The HEART of the MATTER

The African American's Guide to Heart Disease, Heart Treatment, and Heart Wellness

---

The HEART of the MATTER

The African American's Guide to Heart Disease, Heart Treatment, and Heart Wellness

by

HILTON M. HUDSON II, M.D., F.A.C.S.

HERBERT STERN, PH.D.

Hilton Publishing Company • Roscoe, IL

ISBN: 0-9675258-0-2

Notice: The information in this book is true and complete to the best of the author's and publisher's knowledge. This book is intended only as an informative reference and should not replace, countermand, or conflict with the advice given to readers by their physicians. The author and publisher disclaim all liability in connection with the specific personal use of any and all information provided in this book.

Grateful acknowledgment is made to the following for permission to reprint previously published material:

PLUME: Recipes from *Down-home Wholesome* by Danella Carter. Copyright 1995 by Danella Carter. Reprinted by permission of Plume, a division of Penguin Putnam, Inc.

WILBERT JONES: Recipes from *The New Soul Food Cookbook* by Wilbert Jones. Copyright 1996 by Wilbert Jones. Reprinted by permission of author.

Publisher's Cataloging-in-Publication
(Provided by Quality Books, Inc.)

Printed and bound in the United States of America

Contents

ACKNOWLEDGMENTS

My sincere gratitude to these teachers who made my career possible.

Freeman Martin, M.D.
George Rawls, M.D.
John Joyner, M.D.
James Menzoian, M.D.
P. David Myerowitz, M.D.

Promotion of this book is supported, in part, by Pfizer, Inc. whose participation is gratefully appreciated.

Preface

WHAT PATIENTS WANT from doctors is competence and kindness. We trust that you'll find these qualities in this book. But kindness, like love, must sometimes be tough. Here, the toughness is in the facts: African Americans are more likely than whites to die of heart disease. At the same time, kindness insists that this discrepancy in mortality rates is partly within our power to control. By eating well, exercising, and avoiding the substances that abuse the heart, nearly all of us can, in Maya Angelou's phrase, "take our wellness in hand."

This book is our effort to help you do that. We tell you what you need to know about the troubles of the heart, what to do to prevent them, and what to do to recover successfully should you become ill.

This book is addressed to you, the African American woman or man who would rather be healthy than ailing, who would rather stay out of hospitals than stay in them, who would rather live than die. This book is for you, as a person who wants to take charge of your body and your well-being, rather than leave it in the hands of chance and indifference.

We wrote this book as a labor of love. Nothing could reward that labor more generously than for you, individual by individual, to take the book to heart.

Chapter I

AN INTRODUCTION TO CORONARY ARTERY DISEASE

TO BEGIN, WE MUST present some unpleasant but essential facts:

- Coronary artery disease is the number one killer of African Americans.
- African American men develop coronary artery disease earlier than white men.
- African American men with coronary artery disease are more likely to die than white American men who suffer from the same disease.
- African American women with coronary artery disease are more likely to die than white women who suffer from the same disease.
- African American smokers with coronary disease are at higher risk of death than white American smokers with coronary disease.

On the positive side, consider the following:

- African Americans who stop smoking or control their blood pressure decrease their risk of death from coronary artery disease.
- The more you know about coronary artery disease, the better the chances that you and your loved ones won't be killed by it.

Not only is coronary artery disease—also known as cardiovascular disease, or CVD—the leading killer in America but if you're African American the odds are one and a half times greater that you suffer from high blood pressure (or hypertension)—one of the leading risk factors contributing to CVD.

It doesn't have to be this way. A lot of heart disease is preventable and a lot of it is correctable. It can be stopped, or mended, before you suffer a heart attack that will hospitalize you, and, in some cases, kill you. The fact is, what you know won't kill you, and what you don't, will.

Heart disease can often be stopped, or mended, before *you suffer a heart attack.*

Now that you're with us, we'd like to tell you a story.

Though Reverend Asa Johnson had felt poorly for months, he hadn't had much time to think about it. Church membership was falling off and he'd been working twice as hard as ever to turn that around. Worse, for all his efforts there hadn't been much improvement, and some of the members were beginning to blame him.

Through all this Reverend Johnson was troubled by shortness of breath and frequent heaviness in the middle of his chest. Or he'd feel a nagging pain there that spread to his arms or sometimes to his back, and the pain didn't seem to have any connection with what he'd been doing. Sometimes his breath came so hard he wanted to take to his bed. But when these symptoms came, he'd sigh and continue with what he was doing. "At sixty-nine years old," he'd say to himself, "a man's got to expect a few aches and pains. Anyway, I'm a strong black man and a child of the King." As for fatigue, well, he was working hard, but he was working for the Lord, as he'd always done and always would do. This was his life's purpose. For twenty-five years he'd fought with all his heart for the church he served. He couldn't afford to slow down now.

And, after all, he'd taken good care of himself all his life, he never smoked or drank, and he liked to boast, truthfully, that he'd never been sick a day in his life. Yes, he didn't have time for much exercise and he'd put on a few pounds and, yes, his wife thought that he didn't look well and wanted him to see his doctor. But he shook off her insistence, though with his usual patience. Sure, he would go in for an examination, he promised her over coffee one Tuesday morning—he'd go just as soon as he got this trouble at the church settled. She shook her head and said nothing. His health worried her, but he'd never been a man you could talk much sense into about such things.

The next day Reverend Johnson met with his board of directors and the Deacons of his church, hoping that together they could agree on the plan to increase membership that he'd been up several nights thinking and worrying about. So strong was this hope that just before the meeting Reverend Johnson had whispered to himself: "Jesus, stay with me." But twenty minutes into the meeting some of the deacons were fidgeting uneasily. The reverend looked sick. Once he bit his lip, as if he were fighting to keep something back, and his breathing became more and more difficult. Then, as Reverend Johnson, with obvious effort, came to the end of an eloquent appeal for his plan, suddenly and without a sound he fell hard to the floor, unconscious.

He died forty-five minutes later in the emergency room of the community hospital. He'd suffered a massive heart attack.

Consider the following U.S. statistics, posted by the American Heart Association and the American Medical Association:

- One in five males and females have some form of CVD.
- One in three men can expect to develop some major cardiovascular disease before age sixty; the odds for women are one in 10.5.
- More than 2,600 Americans die each day of CVD—an average of one death every 33 seconds.
- CVD claims more lives each year than the next seven leading causes of death combined.
- Since 1900, CVD has been the number one killer in the United States in every year but one (1918).
- Currently, 69 million Americans suffer from cardiovascular disease.
- This year, 1.5 million people will have heart attacks.
- There will be 500,000 deaths among these 1.5 million people.

What happened to Reverend Johnson could obviously have happened to anyone—male or female, black or white. It happens to 2,600 Americans every day, one death every 33 seconds.

Statistics give us the context, but people are more interesting than numbers. So let's take a closer look at what actually happened to Asa Johnson. If Reverend Johnson had seen a doctor in time, he would have learned that his pains, fatigue, and hard breathing pointed to angina. Angina is the body's way of telling us that the heart isn't getting the blood it needs to function normally. And it's marked by the kinds of discomfort Reverend Johnson suffered—that is, a feeling of heaviness, pressure, or pain in the chest, pain that sometimes spreads to the arms or neck or jaw, or radiates to the back.

Angina is the body's way of telling us that the heart isn't getting the blood it needs to function normally.

Angina results from what most of us call hardening of the arteries, and what doctors call arteriosclerosis, or, more simply, coronary artery disease or just plain coronary disease. It's not very different from the kind of plumbing problem you might experience at home when the water flow in the pipe slows or is interrupted by calcium buildup or something that sticks at a bend in the pipe.

In the human body, what clogs the arteries isn't only calcium but also fat deposits. When these clogs or blockages occur in the arteries that feed the heart, because the supply of oxygen to the heart is restricted, symptoms of angina will occur. Like every other organ in the body, the heart needs blood in order to function properly. If the supply of oxygen-rich blood fails, the heart will fail. That failure may be mild or severe, but if the condition

How cholesterol forms on the wall of an artery

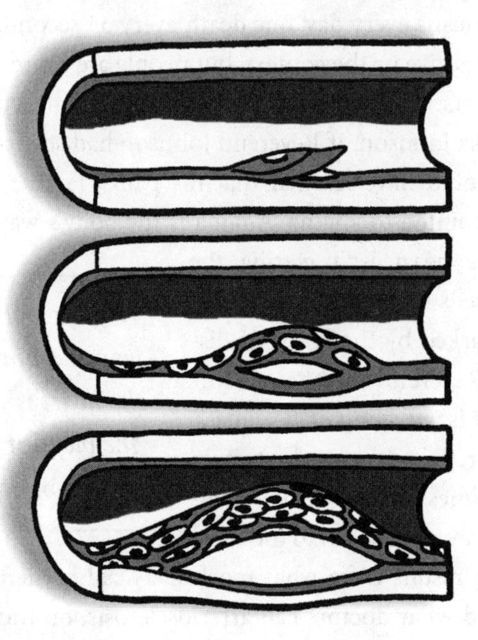

that led to the problem isn't addressed, the heart will become less and less able to do its job, and the symptoms of angina will eventually result in a heart attack.

The heart needs blood in order to function properly. If the supply of oxygen-rich blood fails, the heart will fail

A heart attack occurs when small or large parts of the heart muscle die because they aren't receiving nourishment. In extreme cases, like Reverend Johnson's, the entire heart is affected, and the result is death.

ANATOMY OF A HEART ATTACK

Because we'll return often to the way the heart works when it's well and doesn't work when it's damaged, here's an anatomy lesson about the heart and the circulation system that feeds and flows from it.

You know that the heart is a muscle—*the* muscle. Like all muscles it needs oxygen-enriched blood to function effectively. Deprived of blood, the heart, like any other muscle, suffers. That suffering can be more or less extreme. If the blood flow is decreased so that the heart starves for blood but is still sufficiently alive to function, the condition is called *ischemia,* which simply means a deficiency of blood flow. The more extreme case of heart attack, or *myocardial infarction,* means that the flow of blood has been so impaired that the heart, literally starving for blood, is dying.

Now let's look at this in a little more detail. The heart is divided into four chambers: two upper chambers and two lower ones. The upper chambers are called the *right atrium* and the *left atrium.* The lower chambers are the *right ventricle* and the *left ventricle.* Blood enters the heart through the right atrium. All the blood in the body, from the tip of your toes to the top of your head, usually passes through the right atrium.

From the right atrium, it passes to the right ventricle, the second chamber, where it is pumped into the pulmonary arteries that channel the blood up into the lungs. When we breathe, we take in oxygen that is delivered to the blood pumped from the right ventricle into our lungs. Once that blood, now enriched with oxygen, is ready to leave the lungs, it goes into the third chamber called the left atrium, and from there it goes to the left ventricle. That fourth chamber has the crucial function of pumping the blood into the *aorta*—the major blood vessel coming off the heart that supplies blood to every other artery in the body.

The aorta, because it feeds all these secondary arteries, is responsible for supplying the oxygen-rich blood and nutrients to every organ of the body. It does this by means of branches, the aorta resembling the trunk. The branches, or *arteries*, feed our muscles, tissues, and organs. This is possible through a system of *capillaries,* which are narrower tubes that transfer blood from the organs to their destinations. It is from the capillaries that the muscles, tissues, and organs extract the oxygen and nutrients they need to function properly.

Once that extraction has occurred, the blood travels from capillaries into *veins.* These veins carry the blood to the larger veins called the *superior vena cava* and the *inferior vena cava.* And, if you get the gist, you'll have guessed that those large veins carry the blood back to the first chamber of the heart, the right atrium, where the process begins again.

To review, blood already drained of oxygen and nutrients comes into the heart, where it is resupplied with oxygen, then pumped through the left atrium to the left ventricle, and out through a major highway of the heart—that is, the major artery—called the aorta. The aorta disperses blood throughout the body and into small sidestreets (also called arteries) that deliver blood, by way of capillaries, to the tissues, muscles, and organs. There, the oxygenated nutrients are extracted and the blood is carried through the veins back to the right side of the heart.

There are two last details: first, coming off the aorta are two arteries—the right coronary artery and the left coronary artery.

Decreased blood flow to heart may cause heart muscle damage

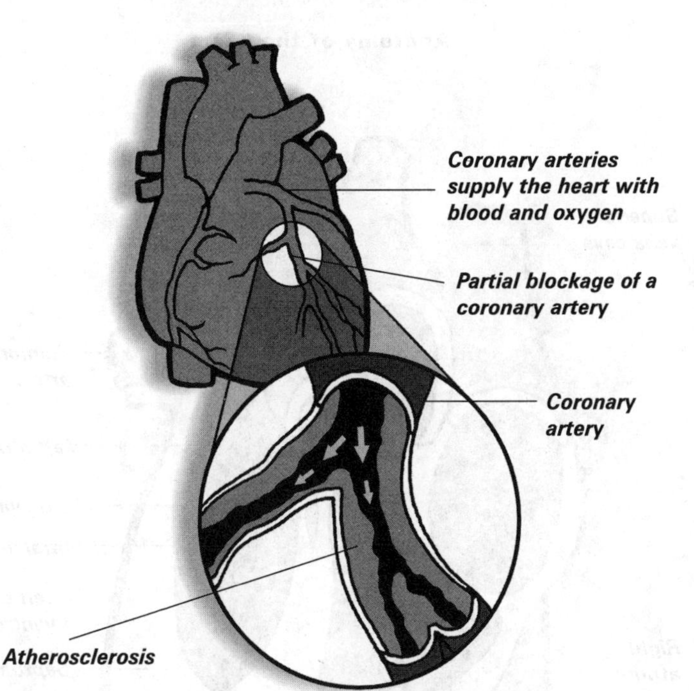

Coronary arteries progressively closing (from left to right) resulting from coronary artery disease.

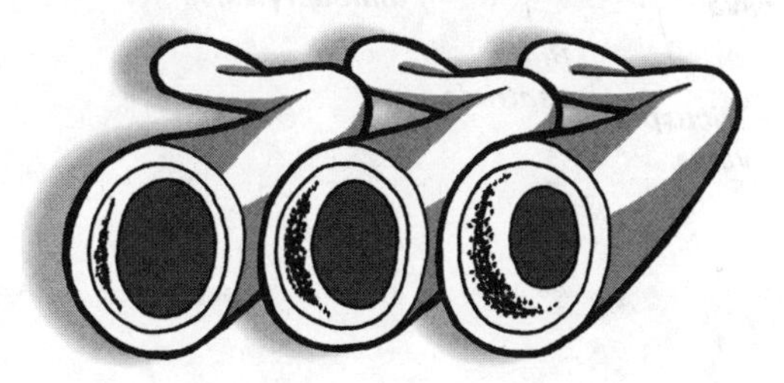

Anatomy of the heart

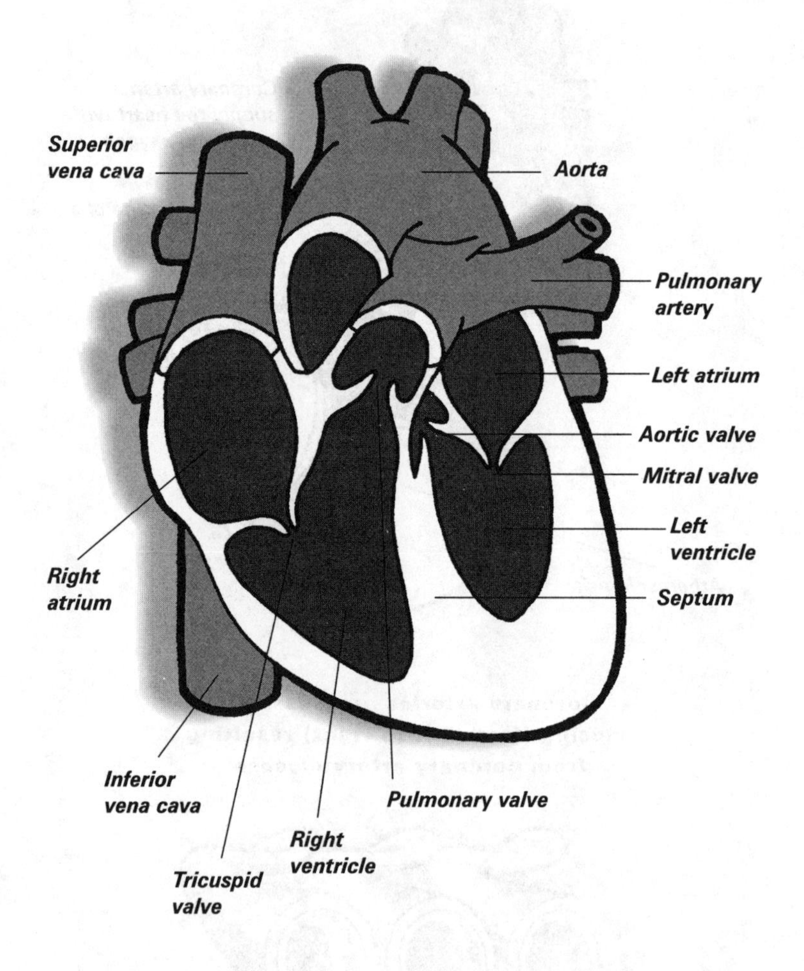

As their names indicate, the right coronary artery supplies the right side of the heart with blood and the left coronary artery supplies the left side of the heart with blood. When these arteries become clogged, the result can be angina or a heart attack.

Second, as the drawing makes clear, the aorta divides into two other arteries called the carotid arteries. When the carotid arteries become blocked, the result will be a stroke.

The good news is that not all, or even most, heart attacks are fatal. If you suffer one, you have a good chance of recovery if you get prompt and appropriate treatment. But, as with other problems, this one is far better nipped in the bud. Once there has been a heart attack, even if it isn't fatal, damage has been done to the heart itself, and repair of, and recovery from, that damage is far more difficult than taking preventive measures to avoid the problem. As to the chances of recovering from a stroke, fully or partially, that depends on how much damage was done. The more serious the stroke, the more likelihood of coma or death. In the case of minor strokes, the chance for recovery is good.

Most heart attacks are not fatal!

RECOGNIZING THE SYMPTOMS OF CORONARY ARTERY DISEASE

Recognizing the symptoms of CAD is the first step toward curing it. In Reverend Johnson's case, these symptoms included:

- Rapid pounding of his heart
- Shortness of breath

- Pain or pressure located in the center of his chest, sometimes spreading to the arms, back, or jaw

Other symptoms include:

- Swelling of the legs
- Fainting spells
- Nausea and vomiting

But even before symptoms are apparent, there's a way of anticipating them. Doctors call such signs *risk factors*—preconditions that make it likely that someone may have a heart attack. Here's a list of risk factors, in a descending order of urgency (which doesn't mean that any should be ignored):

1. High blood pressure (which we discuss in detail in chapter 8)
2. High cholesterol levels (In chapter 12 we talk about the distinction between "good" cholesterol [HDL] and "bad" cholesterol [LDL]. For the time being, when we say "cholesterol," we mean bad cholesterol.)
3. High fat content in diet (see chapters 12 and 13), which may lead to high cholesterol levels and to still another risk factor—that is,
4. Excess weight and diabetes
5. Smoking
6. Advanced age
7. Family history of heart disease
8. Lack of exercise
9. Excessive alcohol use

Look these over. Only two of the risk factors are totally beyond our control. We cannot avoid aging (except by the worse alternative), and we can't unwrite our genetic makeup. We *can* watch what we eat, we can exercise, and thus lower our blood pressure, and we certainly can stop smoking or, even better, never begin. These aren't lifestyle matters—they're matters of life and death.

Before we discuss symptoms further in chapter 2, we want to say a few words about hypertension—high blood pressure—because it's the most dangerous risk factor, especially for African Americans. Elevated blood pressure, no matter how mildly elevated, is likely to result in coronary artery disease. It is one of the body's early warning systems.

HIGH BLOOD PRESSURE AND ITS CONSEQUENCES

Blood pressure is usually reported with a top and bottom number—specifically, the systolic blood pressure is reported first over the diastolic pressure. Don't be put off by the terminology. What it stands for is simple enough. The *systolic blood pressure*—that is, the top number—measures the pressure in the arteries when the heart is beating—that is, contracting. The *diastolic blood pressure*—the bottom number—measures the pressure of the blood in the arteries when the heart is relaxed. Your doctor will tell you that you have hypertension (high blood pressure) if the top number (systolic) is greater than 140 or the bottom number (diastolic) is greater than 90.

Elevated blood pressure, no matter how mildly elevated, is likely to result in coronary artery disease.

How blood pressure is measured

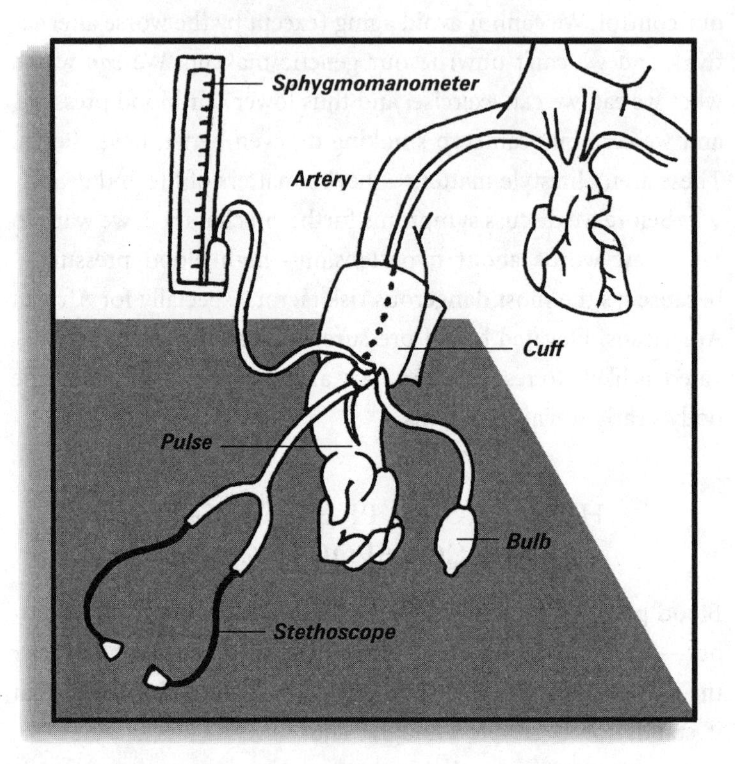

Of the risk factors that threaten African American patients, hypertension is the most common and the most severe. The upside is that it is treatable. To ignore it is to buy serious trouble.

In this case, trouble comes in several forms. The first is coronary artery disease itself. As you know, that means the arteries around the heart are plugged up. The second is congestive heart failure, which means that the heart is overworked and therefore weak. And the third, most sadly, is stroke.

If high blood pressure is treated aggressively and not ignored, the risk of coronary artery disease, congestive heart failure, or stroke is greatly decreased. This may be the most important medical fact in this book, so let us repeat it: *Controlling your blood pressure greatly decreases your risk of suffering coronary disease.*

If high blood pressure is treated aggressively and not ignored, the risk of coronary artery disease, congestive heart failure, or stroke is greatly decreased.

Failure to treat high blood pressure will eventually lead to damage to, and weakening of, the walls of the arteries. These weakened and damaged arterial walls eventually narrow and become clogged with cholesterol, fats, red blood cells, and platelets. Instead of a smooth stream bed, picture a fast-flowing stream whose bed is cluttered with rocks and debris torn loose from the banks and tumbled by the torrent. Bad arteries resemble this type of stream. The higher the blood pressure, the more likely the walls have become damaged, and that damage, with its debris, leads to blood clots and closing of the arteries.

Even mild hypertension needs to be treated. Sometimes that treatment means you need to change your ways—eating differently, cutting down on salt, alcohol, and other substances that make hypertension worse. Sometimes treatment means medicine. But the fact is that hypertension rarely goes away by itself. It's your body's way of saying you need to change your life. We take up this discussion in more detail in chapter 8.

Let's add a word here about congestive heart failure (CHF) and strokes, the other two possible consequences of hypertension. CHF means that the heart is not pumping effectively.

Because it is weak, it can't push blood out of itself in an efficient way and has to work overtime. It must pump more frequently and harder to supply blood and oxygen to the brain. This condition leads to a heart that is overworked and enlarged. Untreated, CHF eventually leads to complete heart failure.

The last of the three major forms of heart trouble is stroke. The carotid arteries carry blood to the brain. If the blood pressure in these carotid arteries is high, the artery walls become weakened and start to close, reducing the oxygen flow to the brain. This decrease of blood flow and oxygen to the brain leads to ministrokes (TIAs or transischemic attacks) or full-blown strokes. And because there's a decrease or stoppage of the blood flow to the brain, the brain itself dies.

High blood pressure is more common in African Americans than in whites and is a leading cause of early morbidity and mortality in the African American population. It doesn't have to be that way. All that's necessary is that we pay attention to what the body tells us and that we know how to get the right treatment.

Chapter 2

THE SYMPTOMS OF CORONARY ARTERY DISEASE

ALEXANDER SAMSON didn't feel well one January morning, but he had his pride. Over coffee he joked to himself: "A man's gotta do what a man's gotta do." And what he had to do that day was take down the Christmas lights from the front of his house.

"Get someone else to do it and you stay here and help me take the tree down and clean up this house," said his wife Judith. But no, he'd rather work outside, and alone.

By the time Alexander had lugged the ladder from the garage to the front of the house, he already was short of breath and felt a heaviness in the middle of his chest. But this was nothing new. He'd been tired a lot lately, and the trouble breathing and pressure in his chest were just part of that. He'd expected a livelier retirement, but he didn't feel like doing very much. Anyway, why should he? He'd worked hard for thirty years. Why run around now? When neighbors or church members or his sons and daughters asked how he was doing, his answer was always the same: "Fine. I'm getting along just fine." And in most respects he was. He'd never had a long illness or had to go to the hospital except for a few stitches to close up a wound he'd gotten at work. And though somewhere down the line a doctor had told him that he had "high blood pressure and a touch of the sugar," he'd never done much about it.

Despite the hard job of lugging the ladder and climbing it, Alexander felt the bitter cold. He hadn't worked long before his chest began to hurt him worse than before and he couldn't catch his breath. He came down the ladder to rest a little, but he wanted to finish the job, and before long he climbed back up, only to feel the same discomfort again, this time more severe.

Now there didn't seem to be any way around it. He went inside to tell his wife what he was experiencing. "Just let me lie down for a minute. I'll be fine." But no, she wouldn't just let him lie down. Instead, she drove him to the local emergency room. Events there moved fast. After the nurse took his blood pressure and listened to his chest, a doctor gave him a more thorough physical examination. "I'm sure you don't enjoy all this fussing over you, Mr. Samson, but we've got to do a couple of tests."

First, there was an EKG—an electrocardiogram—that provided a graphic display of each heartbeat. Then there were blood tests, to determine if Alexander's blood showed traces of the enzymes released by the heart muscle during a heart attack. Finally, Mr. Samson was wheeled to the cardiac catheterization lab, where a cardiologist inserted an intravenous (IV) tube into an artery in his left groin. "This way," the doctor told him, "we can get a picture of the arteries around the heart, to tell if they're plugged up or not. It gives us a kind of roadmap of the arteries that feed the heart blood."

"Oh my Jesus," Mr. Samson said. Despite his discomfort and anxiety, he meant it. He'd been a machinist all his life, and these high-tech gadgets and procedures impressed him.

They impressed his doctor in a different way. The tests revealed that, although Mr. Samson hadn't had a heart attack, the major arteries around his heart were blocked so seriously that he'd likely suffer a heart attack in the next few days if something wasn't done to intervene. That heaviness in the chest and shortness of breath he'd been bothered by were early warning signs. His heart needed more blood than it was getting. Fortunately, in this case Mr. Samson and his wife had listened to the warning signs. Unfortunately, every day hundreds of African Americans die because they ignore these signs.

DON'T IGNORE THE WARNING SIGNS

Every day, across the United States, hundreds of African Americans die simply because they have ignored the warning signs of coronary artery disease (CAD). This is a message that has to be repeated over and over again. And, though we've touched on these signs before, they bear repeating:

- Pain in the center of the chest—or, more commonly, a pressure experienced as a tightening vice, or as an elephant sitting on the chest. This sensation is felt just under the breast bone, sometimes to the left side of the chest under the nipple.

- Sometimes, a persistent pain in the left or right arm. Such feelings of pressure often occur while the victim is exercising, running, or out in the cold working, as Mr. Samson was. The pain can be urgent enough to require the victim to slow down or stop what he or she is doing.
- Any chest pain or pressure that goes down the left arm or up to the throat, or jaw or back, or even to the lower back, and that lasts ten minutes or more.
- Shortness of breath.

While these symptoms are common to most victims of heart disease, regardless of race, studies show that African Americans are less likely to attribute the symptoms to heart problems. True, the symptoms could simply be the result of an especially bad day or plain old age. But wisdom requires that, when the symptoms persist, they be taken seriously. Only a doctor, by an appropriate medical examination, can determine how threatening they are. The sooner the symptoms are addressed, the better the chance of early diagnosis, medical intervention, speedy recovery, and extended life.

African Americans are less likely to attribute the symptoms to heart problems.

Shortness of breath, heavy breathing, and the feeling of being hungry for air mean that the heart isn't doing its job. And there are other signs:

- Swelling of the feet or legs
- Feeling tired all the time and lacking energy
- Loss of appetite

These last signs may be symptoms of Congestive Heart Failure, a condition we will take up in chapter 7. For the moment, it is enough to say that these symptoms of CHF mean your heart isn't pumping as efficiently as it should. It isn't doing its work properly because it isn't receiving the blood it needs. It isn't receiving the blood it needs because the arteries that supply the blood are clogged.

The causes of CHF are various. It can simply be a late stage of coronary disease, or the result of high blood pressure or valve problems in the heart. But it can also be caused by viral or bacterial infection or alcohol abuse.

Coronary blockage

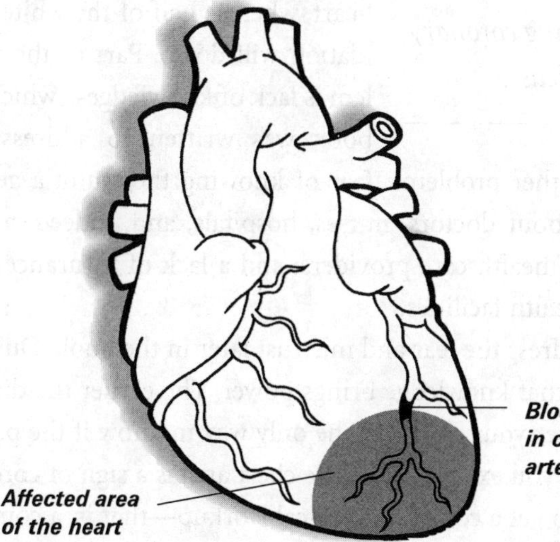

Coronary arteries feed the heart with blood. A blocked coronary, as seen above, will prevent blood from getting to this area of the heart. The heart muscle eventually dies resulting in a heart attack or myocardial infarction (see darkened area to the right).

Its symptoms too can vary. Weight gain, shortness of breath, poor energy, and other unspecific symptoms can be indicators. Unlike coronary disease, CHF does not provide such specific symptoms as chest pain. The essential point is that coronary disease results from a blocked artery or arteries, while CHF means the heart is not working well because some of the heart muscle is dead.

But the most common reason for heart failure is underlying coronary disease, which is ignored by thousands who suffer from symptoms every day, particularly African Americans. Only a third of African Americans who suffer from the symptoms we've described will attribute them to the heart, whereas half of the white population will do so. Part of the problem is lack of knowledge—which this book was written to address. But there are other problems: fear of knowing the truth; a general paranoia about doctors, nurses, hospitals, and, indeed, a deep mistrust of health care providers; and a lack of insurance or of access to health facilities.

The most common reason for heart failure is underlying coronary disease.

We address the fear and mistrust later in the book. Our own attitude is that knowledge brings power. The earlier the diagnosis, the better your chances. The only way to know if the pain or discomfort you experience in the chest area is a sign of coronary disease is to get a complete medical workup—that is, a complete medical examination, including an EKG, a chest x-ray, the appropriate blood or other lab work, and/or invasive or noninvasive cardiac testing. Such a procedure often means the difference between life and death. Lack of knowledge, poor access to health facilities, and paranoia among black Americans—though they can have real social and economic causes—have too often led to inadequate treatment, treatment that comes too late, and deaths that could have been avoided.

Only a third of African Americans who suffer from the symptoms of coronary disease will attribute them to the heart, while half of the white population will.

Let's change that—starting here, starting now. Here's another lesson that could help you to live a longer and more productive life. The heart is a muscular pump that, like all muscles and organs of the body, needs blood to survive. Blood vessels around the heart deliver blood to the heart muscle. When the heart doesn't receive enough blood, heart symptoms occur.

MYOCARDIAL ISCHEMIA

The condition in which the heart doesn't receive enough blood is called *myocardial ischemia.* It occurs when the blood vessels around the heart that feed blood to the heart are clogged or blocked. Untreated myocardial ischemia can play itself out in three phases: *angina* (the general name for the condition in which the heart doesn't get enough blood), *heart attack* (myocardial infarction), and *sudden death.*

In some cases (10 to 20 percent), angina is "silent"—that is, the patient experiences none of the usual symptoms. And angina can be stable or unstable. When it is stable, it is predictable. For example, exertion will always bring pain, and resting will always stop it. Unstable angina is more dangerous. Symptomatic pain may come when the victim is resting, or, if it comes during exertion, it may not go away when the victim is at rest. It is also more likely to lead to a heart attack.

But these distinctions aren't essential to the patient. What is important is that he or she recognize the symptoms and seek appropriate care.

Myocardial ischemia (the condition in which the heart doesn't receive enough blood) can cause a heart attack, as you know. While angina is a symptom that the heart isn't getting enough blood, in the case of a heart attack, the blood flow to the heart stops completely, and the part of the heart affected will die. The death rate for heart attack is estimated to be 8 percent to 10 percent, and may run higher.

Myocardial ischemia can—though only when there are rare complications—cause sudden death, and it's common. The heart goes into a dangerous arrhythmia (irregular beat) and then stops. It is this kind of heart attack that's most publicized by the media, and that's unfortunate. Such episodes happen, certainly, as we saw in the case of Reverend Johnson, but they are relatively rare. The damage done by the wide publicity given to such cases, with all their drama, is that people get a false sense of fatalism. "See, nothing can be done. If it's going to happen, it's going to happen." That's one way we rationalize not taking care of ourselves.

The only *way to know if the pain or discomfort you experience in the chest area is a sign of coronary disease is to get a complete medical workup.*

The truth is that heart attacks usually follow warnings in the form of angina symptoms. And angina, when diagnosed and treated appropriately, usually has a good prognosis.

REVIEW

Let's end this chapter with a review. Answer true or false, then read the last paragraph.

1. Victims of heart disease usually die suddenly with no prior symptoms.
2. If you have coronary artery disease there's nothing you can do about it.
3. Chest pains and discomfort or tightness in the chest are just signs that you're getting older.
4. Feeling tired all the time, or less energetic, is just another sign that you're getting older.
5. Once cardiac symptoms occur, there's nothing you can do to reverse the process.
6. If cardiac symptoms are ignored long enough, they usually go away.

If you answered *false* to all of them, you passed. These are all misconceptions that lead to delay in early diagnosis and treatment. They also lead to countless unnecessary deaths in all Americans, especially African Americans. Sure, it's a misfortune to develop coronary artery disease. But it's a far worse misfortune to ignore symptoms, which, when recognized, can point you toward treatment and recovery. All you have to do is recognize them early.

Chapter 3

MEDICAL TREATMENT OF CORONARY ARTERY DISEASE

We've been talking about what the symptoms of coronary artery disease(CAD) tell you if you listen to them. We haven't said much about what happens after the doctor tells you that you have coronary artery disease. Is surgery the only solution? And, if not, how do you and the doctor choose between treatment options?

Let us introduce you to Bigger Gordon. Bigger has a lot going for him. He's bright, energetic, and takes pretty good care of himself. He doesn't drink, and he plays basketball once a week in his church league. True, he smokes—"a little," according to Bigger, and "a lot," according to his wife. But, he says, his work has its tensions, and cigarettes and an occasional cigar help him to handle stress.

Bigger is a well-educated man who graduated at the top of his class from Hampton University in Virginia, and his life has been good so far. He's an excellent father to his two kids, and he and his wife are the best of companions. As for his job, it's the job he was born for, as he often says. As the first African American to hold the position of vice president of finance in a multi-million-dollar company, he's determined to be better than the best. That means some stress, but he seems to thrive on it. There's nothing Bigger has looked forward to more than going to work each morning.

But all that has changed for Bigger since the spring of 1998, when, after two weeks of slight pressure in his chest, he awoke one morning with alarming chest pain and presented himself for examination at the local emergency room. Bigger had a pretty good idea of what he was in for. Coronary artery disease runs in his family. He saw his mother die from it, and his father became a semi-invalid because of congestive heart disease.

In the emergency room Bigger was put through a full cardiac workup: physical examination, lab work, chest x-ray, and electrocardiogram (EKG). Meanwhile, the emergency doctor called in a cardiologist, who, on the basis of the examination and tests, agreed with the diagnosis of unstable angina.

"Tell you what, Mr. Gordon. Let's do one more test—a coronary angiogram. That'll give us a closer look at the arteries and help us to evaluate any potential damage. From there, we can know better what we have to do."

What the cardiologist, Dr. Schaeffer, came up with wasn't the best of news, but it wasn't the worst either. He found that the main artery that feeds the heart was 20 percent blocked, and there was blockage in several minor arteries. But Dr. Schaeffer didn't recommend surgery. "I think that this can be satisfactorily treated without that," he said.

Bigger took the news with mixed feelings. Nobody loves the idea of going under the knife. At the same time, the analytical part of his mind was uneasy. "Look, Dr. Schaeffer, I certainly don't want surgery if I don't need it, but I need to get this fixed. I don't like the idea of messing around with it for years, waiting for the other shoe to fall. Maybe it would be better to go in and get the whole thing taken care of now—you know, to have the surgery and get this all behind me."

"I'll tell you what, Mr. Gordon. You listen to what I have to say. Then, if you still feel uneasy about my recommendation, we'll call in another cardiologist." Bigger knew how to listen. And what he heard was roughly this:

In a sense, heart issues are lifestyle issues. The way we eat, the way we spend our days, the substances we ingest, the way we manage the inescapable stress in our lives—it all bears on the health of our heart. If all Americans consciously controlled their cholesterol, their blood pressure, their diabetes, if they smoked and drank less and exercised more, coronary artery disease would be much less of a problem than it is.

Much of what hurts the heart is avoidable. And, though most people aren't ready to hear this until after they've had heart trouble, even after the heart has suffered injury it's not too late to change habits, and, by changing them, to help the heart to heal.

The patient is in large part his or her own doctor

The patient is in large part his or her own doctor. For instance, before he even mentioned medication, Dr. Schaeffer told Bigger at once that an essential part of his treatment was to stop smoking. "It's up to you, Bigger," he said. "I can only give you the facts, and the facts are these. Cigarette smoking is dangerous and can be lethal to every organ in the body, and especially to the heart. The chemicals in cigarettes directly cause damage to coronary arteries—damage that will eventually lead to blockage, heart attacks, and strokes.”

The chemicals in cigarettes directly cause damage to coronary arteries—damage that will eventually lead to blockage, heart attacks, and strokes.

“Yeah, well, I don’t want to sound cynical, but what’s the difference now, when the damage has already happened?” Bigger asked.

“Let me give you another fact,” said Dr. Schaeffer. If you keep smoking, whether you are treated medically or surgically, your chance of recovery is decreased. If you have bypass surgery, smoking will lead to premature closure of the bypass grafts and will leave you as bad off as when you started. I know, you hear a lot of people say, smoking’s not the worst thing in the world. They’ll tell you about friends and relatives who lived to be eighty and smoked down to their last day. Sure, it happens. But for every one of those, thousands die of heart attacks or heart failure for which smoking was a primary cause. Those are the facts. You make the choice.”

Okay,” Bigger said. “You’ve convinced me. I’ve always told myself I could quit when I chose to. Now I choose to. But some of this other stuff isn’t under my control. You tell me my blood pressure is high. Well, so was my mother’s and my father’s and their mother’s and father’s before them. Not much I can do about that, is there?”

“I don’t want to sound smug,” Dr. Schaeffer said, “but the answer is: ‘Actually, quite a lot.’ For example, you can exercise.”

"But I do, once a week—basketball in the church league. You should see me go at it. They call me "Air Bigger."

Dr. Schaeffer agreed that was fine. "But it's not enough," he said. He explained that they could bring Bigger's blood pressure down with medication, but it was more important in the long run for Bigger to bring it down by himself.

"I've got patients who swear by meditation. Not only do they swear by it, but as far as I can tell, it works for them. It's one way of getting in touch with the part of yourself that isn't stressed and that doesn't need to run at full throttle all the time.

"We also have to look more closely at your exercise regime. Playing basketball once a week is fine—or was fine—we won't have you doing that until we get your heart in better shape. But the point here is that you need something regular—say three times a week in a gym, with at least 20 minutes of aerobics each time. Regular exercise lowers blood pressure. Once we have you fixed, that's something you need to make time for.

Regular exercise lowers blood pressure and lowers cholesterol

"Your cholesterol is too high. If we don't change that, it won't do us much good to correct the damage that's already been done. For you, high cholesterol means more damage to the arteries."

"So you're going to put me on a diet of fish and broccoli for the rest of my life. Man, that's going to be tough. I love to barbecue on the weekends."

"Nothing that bad. My view is, if you're not eating some of the things you enjoy, you may cut the cholesterol, but you'll add to your stress," explained Dr. Schaeffer. "The diet I'm going to recommend allows you to eat a variety of tasty things, but it requires you to keep mental tabs on how much cholesterol you take in. [The reader can find out more about this diet in chapter 13.]

"I'm not saying that this isn't a drag. We all want to eat what we want to eat when we want to eat it. But you've got to think about the trade-off. What you're going to find, Bigger, is that, if you stick to the regime we're plotting out here, you'll feel better than you have for years.

"I have to say that for you it isn't all going to be lifestyle remedies. Your blood pressure is too high, and we have to address this immediately. For a while, at least, I'm going to put you on medication. Then, when we lower your blood pressure to where it should be, we'll see if we can gradually control it without medication.

"My guess is that if you watch what you eat, stop smoking, get into a regular exercise routine, and, if it suits you, some meditation as well, we can get you in reasonably good shape. I don't want to kid you on this. You do have coronary artery disease, and nothing can make it entirely undone. But we can have you living a healthy, normal life, and playing as much basketball as you want, but you have to stick to the plan we've talked about here.

"Let me sum this all up. You have coronary artery disease that your smoking and high blood pressure have contributed to. I'm going to treat this in two ways. First, I'll give you medication, nitroglycerin, that will help increase the blood flow to your heart when your heart is stressed. It does that by opening up the arteries around the heart whenever the heart needs extra blood.

"I'm also going to put you on medication to help control your blood pressure. [The reader can find out more about high blood pressure, also called hypertension, in chapter 8.] But, as I've said, medication can't do the whole job. You have to support it. And you do that by, first, not smoking; second, by exercising three times a week; third, by keeping your weight down; and, fourth, by eating low-fat and low-sodium foods. You'd be surprised at how tasty and varied such a diet can be—and I speak from experience. And on Sundays I'll give you time off for good behavior and you can barbecue and eat what you want, but in moderation.

"You stick to this plan and we'll stop the progression of your coronary artery disease—maybe we'll even reverse some of it. I'd like you to make an appointment for a month from now. At that time, I'll examine you and check your blood pressure and cholesterol levels, and we'll see if you're really in shape, Air Bigger." Dr. Schaeffer smiled at Bigger.

Bigger was lucky in one respect. He didn't have a serious weight problem and he knew something about exercise. What if he hadn't? Dr. Schaeffer would have told him much the same thing, but he might have had a harder time convincing him. Excess weight, or obesity, which is disproportionately high among African Americans, and especially among African American women, is a major risk factor in matters of the heart. Often, overweight people have stopped exercising, or never did exercise.

Excess weight, or obesity, disproportionately high among African Americans, and especially among African American women, is a major risk factor in matters of the heart.

THE IMPORTANCE OF EXERCISE

Exercise is an essential part of heart treatment. Exercising regularly lowers blood pressure and cholesterol. It lowers cholesterol by allowing your body to metabolize it more effectively—that is, to burn it off. We often forget that the heart is a muscle and that it needs exercise just as other muscles do in order to remain efficient and strong.

Excess weight means more work for your heart—more wear and tear. Talk to anyone who works out at a gym or at home about how exercise lowers stress levels. Life is stressful, and it can be especially stressful for African Americans. Although we can't always eliminate the causes of stress, we can do something about the effects. In chapters 5 and 10, we describe exercise routines that are easy, fun, and that relieve stress and bring about the other good things we've described.

> *Life is stressful, and especially so for African Americans. But, while we can't always eliminate the causes of stress, we can do something about the effects.*

Maybe you're going to tell us that you know lots of people who exercise regularly and still have heart attacks. Maybe you even remember the famous Flo Jo, who died of a heart problem despite being in ultimate shape. It's true: Life isn't always fair, and life isn't always consistent. We know a lot about the heart, but mysteries remain.

What isn't a mystery are the odds. For every ten people who keep in shape and nevertheless die of heart disease, thousands die due to lack of exercise, and because they don't control their cholesterol and blood pressure levels. You're smart enough to play the odds.

Exceptional cases like that of Flo Jo aside, if you have a strong heart as a result of exercise and conditioning, even if you have the misfortune to suffer a heart attack, your chances of surviving are greatly increased. Do you want to live longer and live better? Play the odds.

NONSURGICAL TREATMENTS

Now let's look at a slightly different angle. Because Dr. Schaeffer doesn't consider Bigger's condition immediately threatening, and because Bigger is a cooperative and smart patient, the doctor has decided to begin treatment with methods that aren't invasive. If after a few months the improvement isn't what Dr. Schaeffer has hoped for, he still has several resources he can turn to instead of surgery.

There are several non-surgical treatments for coronary disease including angioplasty, stenting of an artery, atherectomy (unplugging an artery).

Remember that coronary disease means that the arteries are clogged and therefore the heart isn't getting enough oxygen–rich blood. Whatever the treatment, it must address that basic problem. In the case of a patient for whom exercise, diet, and stress-relief measures don't bring about the necessary improvements or stability, there remain several options for nonsurgical treatment. These include angioplasty, stenting of an artery, and atherectomy.

Angioplasty

The most common of the treatments we've named is *angioplasty.* It's an outpatient procedure—that is, you usually go home the

A plugged coronary artery being opened via angioplasty

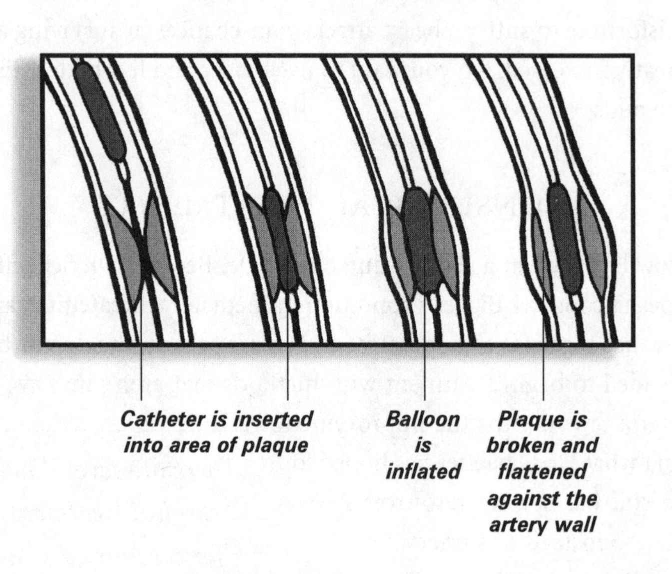

same day the procedure is performed or the next morning—performed by a cardiologist, in the cardiac catheterization lab of a hospital.

The procedure itself begins with the insertion of a small wire, called a catheter, into the blocked coronary arteries. A balloon is attached to the end of the catheter and the catheter is advanced into the arteries that surround the heart. The cardiologist can monitor the progress of the catheter on a TV screen called a fluoroscope. With the heart and the blood vessels that surround it always in view, the cardiologist steers the balloon to the center of the blocked artery. Then the balloon is inflated, causing the blocked vessel to reopen.

How does the catheter find its way to the blood vessels of the heart? Well, it's a little bit like following the yellow brick road. The catheter is inserted in any large blood vessel—usually in the groin area—that leads to the heart. From there, the catheter just follows the path back to the heart.

Angioplasty is usually recommended for patients who have one, or sometimes two, severely blocked coronary arteries. It is also performed in situations where, for whatever reason, heart surgery is considered dangerous or impractical. Generally, angioplasty is painless and straightforward. The patient is mildly sedated with a local anesthetic (that is, the area to be treated is numbed, just as it is in your dentist's office). Angioplasty is a common procedure, performed in university hospitals, teaching hospitals, and community hospitals all over the country.

Naturally, in this treatment as in all medical treatments, there can be a downside. In this case, the risk is that the blood vessel that's been opened can close again, or the blood vessels can tear open (rupture). You can play a significant part in raising your odds of having a successful procedure by finding out as much as you can about the product, which, in this case, is your doctor's competence and experience, and the reputation of the hospital in which the procedure will be performed.

Ask your doctor how many angioplasties he's done and just what his or her success rate is.

You need to ask your doctor how many angioplasties he or she has done and the success rate of these procedures. Don't be embarrassed. You have an absolute right to know. So ask the following questions, politely but firmly, and expect answers:

- How many angioplasties have you personally performed?
- In what percentage of the angioplasties you perform do the arteries close again?
- What is your success rate?
- What happens if the angioplasty doesn't work?
- What complications are possible, and how do you deal with them?

Most well-trained board-certified cardiologists will have no trouble answering these questions freely and openly. If your doctor is defensive, refuses to answer your questions, or seems offended, that should raise a red flag. You need to do what you can to keep the communication going, and that means asking the questions again, if necessary, in the most friendly and unthreatening way you can. If you still don't get a satisfactory response, you'd be wise to refuse the procedure with that particular cardiologist. You can find a better one, more open to his or her patients, more likely to win your confidence. You want no less. After all, next to God, the cardiologist is the person who will carry your life in his or her hands.

If you don't get adequate responses from your physician, you'd be wise to refuse the procedure with that particular doctor.

Stenting

A second nonsurgical procedure for opening blockages in a vessel, and which is used in conjunction with angioplasty, is *stenting.* A stent is a very small coil that keeps a blood vessel open once it has been cleared by angioplasty. The cardiologist first locates the "culprit" artery—the one where the trouble is. He or she opens that vessel with an angioplasty procedure. The cardiologist then inserts the stent. It's that simple. Although the results vary, depending on the extent of the damage and on the cardiologist's experience, in general, angioplasty with stents works even better than angioplasty alone.

Atherectomy

Finally, your cardiologist may suggest, rather than angioplasty or stenting, a procedure called *atherectomy.* Here, a small device is inserted into the blocked artery and cuts through the blockage. Atherectomy is only performed by the most experienced cardiologists and, in general, it's less effective than angioplasty or angioplasty with a stent.

GETTING THE MOST OUT OF PROCEDURES

The procedures that we've been discussing are usually performed in cases where only one or two arteries are blocked, though there are exceptions. It's important for you to realize that such procedures are palliative—that is, they relieve the condition, they avoid heart surgery, but they do not free the patient of coronary artery disease. These procedures are more likely to be effective when patients are ready to take charge of their own destiny by giving up cigarettes, by exercising daily, by reducing stress when possible, and by learning better methods of stress management. And, of course, lowering cholesterol is important.

Even under the best of circumstances, these procedures require, before you submit to them, that you talk openly with your doctor about an alternative plan. Once again, if the doctor is offended or evasive in response to such questions, or if you have the impression that the doctor is too busy to answer your questions, you may need to find another doctor. Again, it's your job to be courteous, open, and nonthreatening. It's the doctor's job to give you all the information you ask for.

It's true that some patients don't want to know. But if you were one of them, you wouldn't be reading this book. In general, the better informed you are about a procedure and about what may follow, the less worried and the less anxious you'll be. And the less worried you are, the better for your heart.

One patient who had refused angioplasty treatment later explained: "It wasn't that I didn't want the angioplasty. But the doctor seemed in such a big hurry, like I wasn't important to him. I guess I was just scared. I wish I had asked more questions." Take those words to heart. If things are moving faster than you're comfortable with, slow them down. Ask your questions. (You'll find more on this subject in Appendix 1, "Your Rights as a Patient.")

Procedures involving the heart—coronary bypass surgery, angioplasty, stenting, or atherectomy—can be stressful and even scary. Ease your mind by asking questions and gaining knowledge. Besides relaxing you and relaxing your doctor, this tactic lets the doctor know that, as an inquiring and informed patient, you have high expectations of him or her and of the hospital.

Chapter 4

CORONARY BYPASS SURGERY

GENERATIONS OF STRONG and successful African American men and women can testify that faith in God and a solid understanding and knowledge of the matter at hand can conquer any fear and move any mountain. In matters of heart surgery, the more you understand in advance, the better. At the same time, on the surgical table, faith—whether faith in the Lord or faith, through knowledge, in the surgical procedure itself—can move mountains.

Naturally, when it comes to having somebody cut you open to repair parts of your body that have never seen the sun, you may not be up to hearing a lot about it in advance. In fact, the moment you learn your heart is in trouble is likely to be one of the toughest experiences you ever have to go through. It's a moment when everything starts moving very fast, as your ordinary life comes to a screeching halt.

Trouble can come in a rush. Bertha Turner had been busy cooking her traditional Sunday dinner, looking forward to the gathering of children and grandchildren. It was the high point of her week. As always, she was doing it all herself, though her daughter and daughter-in-law asked every week if they could come over to help her. "Honey," Bertha would always say, "when I can't cook Sunday dinner without help from my children, well, that's the time for me to check into the rest home." When she put it like that, the younger women just had to let her have her way.

But that Sunday the same old pressure and tightness in her chest that she never talked about to anyone was back—so bad that she had to lie down. When her husband found her, he said, "Girl, something's the matter for sure if you're not in the kitchen at 3:30 on a Sunday."

"Nothing's the matter," Bertha said, more worried about him than she was about herself. "Just that I feel a little tired and my breathing's not what it ought to be. Maybe, just to be safe, you can drive me to the hospital for them to take a quick look. Anyway, everything's in the oven. No need to call the children. We'll be back before they get here."

Once they arrived in the emergency room, you know the drill. The ER (emergency room) physician examined her, called in a cardiologist , and ordered blood work and an EKG (electrocardiogram). All this was happening quickly, and by now Bertha knew that she wouldn't be home for her Sunday dinner. It didn't take long for the tests to clinch that.

It was the cardiac catheterization that told the cardiologist, Dr. Brenner, what he had to do. That test, a dye study of the heart, showed that all the major blood vessels were blocked. Dr. Brenner showed the films to Mr. and Mrs. Turner. "What these pictures say to me," he told them, "is what you must suspect already. You need surgery, Mrs. Turner, and, though I wish this weren't so, I can't give you a lot of time to think about it. If we don't do the surgery, you're going to have a heart attack. That's clear. That's what you've been feeling—angina is the heart's way of warning that it needs attention quickly. If you need to think about it, I can give you until tomorrow morning. All I can say is that there's no doubt in my mind. Any heart doctor looking at these pictures would tell you the same thing I'm telling you."

The Turners looked at the surgeon for a minute or two, unable to speak. Then Bertha broke the silence:

"What are my chances of getting through the operation?"

"Ninety-five percent, Mrs. Turner, if I want to be conservative," Dr. Brenner replied. "But to tell you the truth, I'd put it closer to 98 percent."

"Well, that's good," Mr. Turner said. "Those are good odds."

But Mrs. Turner wanted time to think. "Odds are for horseraces," she said. "If you don't mind my asking, Dr. Brenner, could you tell me how many of these operations you've done and how they came out?"

Dr. Brenner told her, and then he explained the complications that could arise—that is, he gave her a glimpse of what could go wrong and what could possibly put her in that frightening 2 to 5 percent.

"You come back in the morning," she told the doctor, "and I'll be ready to talk."

But when Dr. Brenner left, she turned to her husband and said, "They're not doing any heart surgery on me. I'm putting my life and heart in God's hands only."

It was her daughter who finally persuaded her to have the surgery. “The Lord helps those who help themselves, Mama, and if you don’t let them do this operation, you’re not helping yourself.”

When Dr. Brenner arrived in the morning, Mrs. Turner said, “Okay, then, you do what you have to do.” And her husband put his head down in relief.

“Tell you what,” Dr. Brenner said. “They’ll be here to get you ready in about an hour. If you’d like, I could come in just a little before that and you and I and your family could pray for your good recovery and my best skill. How about that?” That’s what they did an hour later. They made a circle and prayed to the Lord to take good care of Bertha and to guide the surgeon’s hand. And Bertha added a prayer that the Lord take care of her family if she didn’t make it through the surgery.

Before it was over, Dr. Brenner had pretty much remade the arterial pathway that fed Bertha’s heart—a coronary bypass times five (that is, five bypass grafts)—with no complications. Mrs. Turner was home, though not quite ready to cook, in five days. Looking back a year later, during a checkup, she told Dr. Brenner that, although she’d been scared to death, she was grateful to him for a second chance at life.

“It’s been better than the first,” she said. “And I’ll tell you the truth, looking back—it wasn’t half as bad as I’d feared.”

“You’d be surprised how many patients tell us that,” Dr. Brenner said.

USEFUL QUESTIONS TO ASK BEFORE UNDERGOING SURGERY

Let's look at some of the questions that cross a person's mind when he or she is first told heart surgery should be considered.

- Is surgery really necessary?
- Why do I need surgery when other people have angioplasty?
- What will happen if I decide to delay surgery?
- Am I strong enough to undergo surgery?
- Might the surgery itself increase my risk of heart attack?
- How bad will it hurt?
- How long will I be laid up?
- What can I do afterward?
- When can I go back to work?
- Will I be on permanent disability?
- Just how did this happen to me, when I've always watched my weight and diet and taken good care of myself?
- How complicated is this surgery?

Heart surgeons hear these questions often. But these questions too often, out of fear and uncertainty, remain unasked. And sometimes, we're sorry to say, as a result of the doctor's haste or indifference, they remain unanswered. So, while we have Dr. Brenner around, let's talk to him, patient to doctor, and see what we can learn. We're going to imagine you as the patient.

DIALOG WITH DR. BRENNER

Patient: Please tell me why I need this coronary bypass operation, Dr. Brenner. Also, tell me what you're going to be fiddling with, while you're working inside me.

Dr. Brenner: Let's start from scratch. The purpose of the operation is to improve the blood flow to the heart. By doing that, we also decrease angina pains, decrease the chance of a heart attack, decrease the chance of congestive heart failure, and, above all, decrease the chance that the heart will stop suddenly—which, of course, can mean instant death. So, by increasing the blood flow to your heart, we give you a chance for longer life and, at the same time, we ease your fear of sudden heart attack.

The basic idea is to build a bridge around the blocked artery or arteries. In effect, we give the blood new channels to the area of the heart that has been deprived. The bypass graft simply provides a path around the blocked artery.

Patient: Can you tell me exactly how you're going to bring about all these good things?

Dr. Brenner: Sure. The basic idea is to build a bridge around the blocked artery or arteries. In effect, we give the blood new channels to the area of the heart that has been deprived. The bypass graft simply provides a path around the blocked artery.

Patient: I'm interested in the mechanics of this. You know, I feel a little like a broken watch who's talking to the watchmaker. I mean, I have a real interest in the parts you're going to put in and how you're going to rig them.

Dr. Brenner: Sure you do. It's your body. Well, here's a comforting fact to start with. It stays your body. To be sure, we'll need to help it a little while you're under anaesthesia—for instance, with a ventilator that helps you breathe. But the material for the bypass path (sometimes we call it a "tunnel") is one of your own veins. Usually we take it from the leg. Once I have the vein, I attach one end to the aorta—that's the body's biggest artery—which carries blood from the left ventricle of the heart to all the organs.

Then I fasten the other end of the bypass graft to the coronary artery—just past the blockage. So there we have the bypass. Now blood can flow easily past the blockage into the coronary arteries, to feed the heart the nourishment it needs in order to function properly.

Bypass Surgery

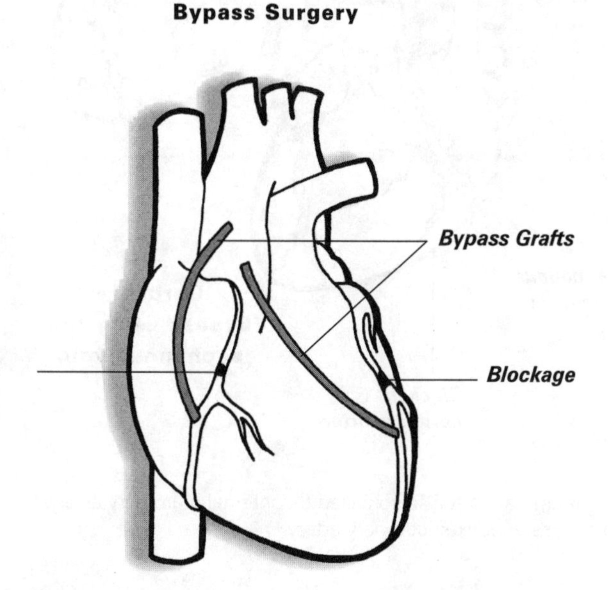

After a typical bypass operation, oxygenated blood bypasses the blockage in the coronary thereby feeding the heart with needed blood.

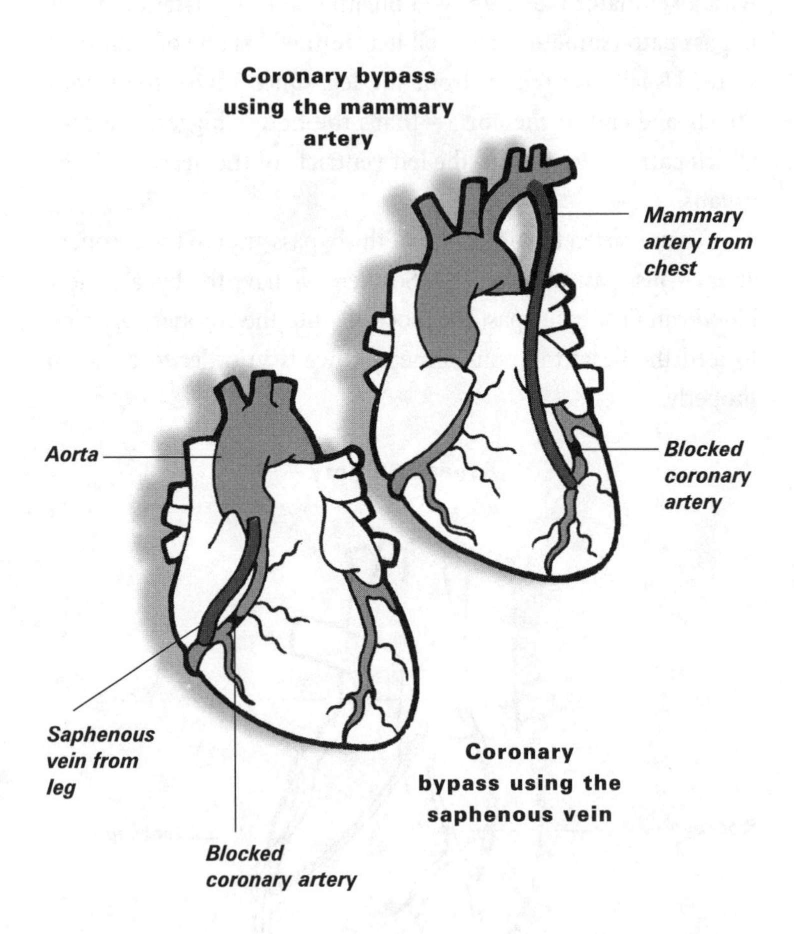

The mammary artery, also called the internal mammary artery, can be used to bypass a blocked coronary artery.

Patient: Okay, that seems clear enough. Now maybe you can help me with this. When people talk about triple and quadruple bypasses, exactly what's that all about?

Dr. Brenner: Well, the principle of the bypass operation is simple enough: to bypass what's severely blocked. If two arteries are blocked, that usually means a two-way bypass; if three, a three-way bypass is usual. The more major arteries are blocked, the more bypasses I must do. But I bypass only seriously clogged arteries, and then, only if they are major arteries.

If two arteries are blocked, that means a two way bypass, if three, a three way bypass.

Patient: Yeah, well, that brings it down to earth. When some friend wants to talk to me about their bypass operation, I guess part of me just doesn't want to know too much. It's as if by keeping ignorant I keep that bad luck away from my door.

Dr. Brenner: Well, I can understand that. When we're afraid of something, we try to block it out, so we won't worry about it. But look—I'm trying to be frank here. I wouldn't want you to think that there was nothing to be scared of. You came to me because you were experiencing the symptoms a heart sends out when it isn't working properly. That's obviously something to take very seriously indeed. Now I'm recommending to you an operation that will probably make your heart work better and make your life safer. But let's say, to use the national average, there's 2 to 5 chances in 100 that I'll fail—that is, that your heart will fail while I'm working on it. Finally, as if that's not enough to think about, even if, as I expect and believe, everything goes well, I wouldn't want you to think that your heart will be as good as new. It won't be. It should be a lot better than it was when I first saw you. That's all I can promise. That's all I can try for.

Let's step out of the dialog for a moment. You're going to need a little time to take in what Dr. Brenner just said, and, as the case of Bertha Turner makes clear, often that's all you get—a little time. How you take in the information will depend on who you are. Calm and wise people react one way; impatient people react another way. There are macho ways and sincerely pious ways, selfish and generous ways, to respond to this situation. You'll find your own because you must. We can hope and pray that we have wisdom and courage to handle this situation. Let's go on.

Patient: Dr. Brenner, I'm as ready as I'll ever be. I've talked it over with my husband and my older son and we've agreed that I need to get this thing done. My next question is, What's the drill? What should I expect between now and the time I wake up in the recovery room?

Dr. Brenner: I've scheduled the operation for the day after tomorrow, at seven in the morning. If the operation were later, I'd ask you to come in that morning. As it is, I'd like you to come in at one o'clock tomorrow afternoon. That gives us time to run a few last-minute tests and to provide some presurgical teaching. But I'm going to work some of that teaching into the discussion we're having now. Ready?

Patient: Sure. I'm going to be your best student.

Dr. Brenner: Okay. Practices will vary a little from one doctor to the next, but here are the basics. I'll have an electrocardiogram run on you, just to make sure that there have been no significant changes in your heart rhythm and heartbeat. I'll also have another chest x-ray done, to make sure your lungs are clear and there aren't any abnormalities there. I don't want any surprises in the operating room.

We also need to type and cross your blood—that is, to make sure we get a safe blood match, because you may need transfusions during the operation, and sometimes we get the blood from the blood bank, where we know that it's been tested and is safe. But, as a double precaution, we prefer to collect your own blood that is lost during the operation with what's called a "cell saver." We then give it back to you in the operating room after the operation is over.

Patient: You guys are really into recycling, aren't you?

Dr. Brenner: Yes, we are. We want to keep your body as close to the original model as we can. But let me tell you a little more about the blood tests. They will also tell us your electrolyte count—electrolytes are chemicals in the blood that keep your cells healthy—and let us check out your nutritional status. One of the blood tests will tell us if your red blood cell count is high enough to allow you to undergo surgery.

Another kind of test is a pulmonary function test—that is, a lung test. It tells the doctor how well you breathe.

Another kind of test we'll have performed—and it's a very important one—is a pulmonary function test—that is, a lung test. We need to know how well you breathe—whether you have any lung problems. If you do, the operation becomes a little more dangerous. An odd fact—don't ask me to explain—is that African Americans who smoke fare worse after surgery than do white Americans who smoke.

Before I operate, I'll give you the results of all these tests. I feel best entering an operation when the patient knows what I know. That way, though of course you'll be unconscious, it's more like a cooperative venture. And, after all, that's what it really is—you and I together working to give you a new chance at life.

Your medical history, including a complete list of medications, your insurance card, and your living will or power of attorney if you have prepared those will be requested.

Patient: Okay. I like the feel of that. Are we ready to go, then?

Dr. Brenner: Just a few more things. We need to have your medical history, including a complete list of medications, your insurance card, and your living will or power of attorney if you have prepared these documents. If you feel too upset to manage these details, ask a loved one to take care of them for you. In any case, they're essential.

Patient: I guess I can take care of all that, or my husband will help me with it. I also wanted to ask you what I should do about the medications I'm on already.

Dr. Brenner: Good question. I need to review these with you. In most cases, I'll want you to continue taking what you're on. If you take aspirin or other blood-thinning medication, I need to know. Aspirin, or medicines like Coumadin, Motrin, or Advil, will increase your bleeding because they tend to "thin" your blood. Therefore, I'll have you stop taking these medications two to seven days before surgery. We don't want your blood so thin that excessive bleeding during surgery might result.

Patient: Well, I feel like I'm about to take a big journey. There's so much to prepare that I'll need a checklist.

Dr. Brenner: Yes, it is a journey, and the more careful we are about details, the more confident we can be that you'll get where you want to go. So here's a few more items for the checklist. I don't want you to eat anything after midnight the day before surgery. As you probably know, if your stomach is full of food when you go under anesthesia, you could vomit. That's bad enough, but what makes it worse is that you could aspirate food down your trachea—that is, your breathing tube—and this could lead to pneumonia and further complications during and after surgery.

Patient: Okay. After that little speech I don't think I'm likely to feel hungry the night before. Anything else?

Dr. Brenner: Well, yes. Since you're a patient who wants to know, there are a few more details I can prepare you for. I'd like you to take a long shower the night before surgery—say, 10 minutes—paying especially careful attention to your chest, the inside of your thighs, and your groin. That shower will lessen the chance of infection, and it's particularly important if you are diabetic and get infections easily.

Patient: I'm not, but I'll shower anyway.

Dr. Brenner: Good. By the way, leave at home personal items that might get lost. And—forgive me if this sounds silly—know the exact time when you're due in the hospital and don't be late. You may not believe this, but I've had patients fail to show up, then tell me they forgot.

Patient: I'll be sure to put it in my appointment book.

Dr. Brenner: Great. I know I'm asking you to take in a lot and to think about things that aren't easy to think about. But it's my view—and my experience confirms it—that the more you know beforehand, the less anxious and frightened you'll feel at the time of the operation. Frankly, that strengthens your chances of survival. And I want you to do whatever will help you relax during this nerve-wracking but unavoidable procedure. If having a picture of a loved one helps you, bring it. Or a bit of scripture. Some people bring calendars as a reminder of when their normal lives will resume. Some people bring a favorite book or one they're looking forward to reading. Or the Bible.

Time for a breather. While reading this isn't quite the same thing as getting ready for surgery, we've tried to make it as close as possible. That means it puts strain on you—no way around that. So take a break and go out and smell the flowers. Brew yourself a cup of coffee—or, as your heart would prefer, something without caffeine such as noncaffeinated tea. Try, as some Buddhists advise, to empty your mind. Then, when you're refreshed, come back to us. Let's continue the conversation with Dr. Brenner.

Dr. Brenner: If you feel comfortable, I'm going to talk to you about the operation, but in more detail than I have earlier. I'm going to walk you through it, so to speak.

Patient: Yes. I'm ready.

Dr. Brenner: First, the anesthesiologist will stop in to see you some time before the operation. She'll explain her part in the operation. Take that visit as another opportunity to ask questions. Be very direct. If you don't understand something, say so. Ask again until the answer is crystal clear in your mind.

What the anesthesiologist will tell you is roughly this: In the operating room, she will give you a sedative and will place monitoring devices on you so that we can monitor your heart and lung functions throughout the surgery. She will continue to give you anesthesia as you deeply sleep.

In the operating room you will receive a sedative. Monitoring devices will be placed on you so doctors can monitor your heart and lung functions throughout the surgery.

Patient: And I suppose you'll now tell me what I'm missing while I sleep through the action?

Dr. Brenner: Exactly. This is the heart of the matter, if you'll forgive the pun. First, the surgical assistants clean your body with an antiseptic solution, and then they drape your chest and leg in sterile drapes, in order to isolate these areas.

Now the operation begins. I start by making a small incision in your chest and an incision in one leg. Next, using a small electric saw, I cut through your breast bone in order to expose your heart. Once I've finished these preliminaries, I connect your heart to the heart-lung machine, or the bypass machine. Its job, in a nutshell, is to do the work of your heart and lungs.

Blood is pumped through a large tube placed in one chamber of the heart. The machine feeds oxygen into the blood; the oxygenated blood is returned to the heart's major artery, the aorta, and then circulates through the body, as it normally does.

The cardiac surgeon helps to regulate this process so that gradually the heart's work is passed on to the machine and the heart itself can be slowed, then actually brought to a standstill.

Patient: Ah. I see that to this point you've just been preparing to operate.

Dr. Brenner: That's exactly right. It's only when the heart is stopped—we stop it mainly by cooling it—that I can get down to the actual work of inserting the bypasses, as I've already described to you. (The machine itself will be operated by a profusionist who works hand in hand with me during the operation.) Once I'm finished with that, we let the heart gradually resume its beat and its normal function. (It does that naturally as it rewarms.) When I'm satisfied that everything, including the bypasses themselves, is working as it should be, I disconnect the heart from the bypass machine and close up the breast bone with wires that will stay there permanently.*

Patient: Listening to all this I'm beginning to feel like a stuffed turkey.

Dr. Brenner: Yeah, a little like that, if you can imagine the turkey not only stuffed but repaired.

Patient: Are we there yet?

Dr. Brenner: Hang on for just a little bit longer. I have to insert a couple of tubes into the chest above the heart in order to drain the blood that accumulates after surgery—ordinarily a very small amount. We're usually able to take these tubes out within a day or two of the surgery. Now we're more or less there.

Patient: And exactly where is "there"?

Dr. Brenner: After the actual surgery, for a few hours we have you in intensive care, where we can monitor you. Between 4 and 7 hours after surgery, you'll wake up. Then we'll remove from your breathing pipe—called the trachea—the breathing tube we inserted just before you went to sleep. At that point—a beautiful moment for everyone—you can talk to your loved ones.

Patient: I suppose I'll be pretty weak and sedated for a while.

Dr. Brenner: Yes, and a bit uncomfortable. But as you probably know, we don't let you stay like that for very long. In the old

---

* Conventional bypass surgery is done this way. Beating heart surgery (also called off-pump surgery) allows us to do bypass surgery while the heart still beats without the use of the heart-lung machine.

days, a patient might lie around for a week or more before beginning to move around and walk. By that time, she would have lost a lot of the strength she came in with. Now we find that we get much better results when we have you not only talking but walking within twenty-four hours after surgery. At the same time, we'll give you all the pain medicine you need to keep you comfortable during the first and second day after surgery. Within three to five days after surgery, you'll go home, unless there are complications.

Within three to five days after surgery you'll go home, unless there are complications.

Patient: So that's it?

Dr. Brenner: Pretty much. That's the standard procedure, anyway. Each surgeon may have his or her own variations. And there have been some major breakthroughs in cardiac surgery. For example, we're beginning to do bypass surgery without splitting the breast bone. And, still more recently, we have found it possible to operate without the use of the heart-lung machine. But, again, the conventional practice is as I described it. Your surgeon is the only one who can decide whether one of these new procedures is appropriate to your case.

You'll understand that, like specialists in any field, we're always trying to find ways to do the job better. But the job itself—to bring oxygen-rich blood to the heart by bypassing the clogged arteries—that is unlikely to change much in the near future.

Patient: As much as I'd like to think that the story ends here, and we all live happily ever after, I need to ask you about something that bothers me. I guess I'll just ask you directly: You've done the operation, you've reduced my chances of suffering a heart attack, and you've relieved my anxiety. But are the repairs permanent?

Dr. Brenner: That's a good question. And I'll answer it as directly as I can: probably. You have an 80 to 85 percent chance of never needing surgery again, which leaves you with a 15 to 20 percent chance that you will need another surgery if the bypass starts to close. You can help yourself by never smoking. If you smoke, the grafts will close earlier. By exercising, watching your diet, keeping your cholesterol and blood pressure controlled, and keeping your weight down, you can help keep your new bypass grafts open. That is, you can play an active role in prolonging your life.

Patient: Okay, I can live with that, if you'll pardon the expression. But I have another fear—I mean, another question. I might not get through the operation—isn't that true?

Dr. Brenner: Yes, I'm sorry to say that it is, although, given your general condition, the odds are excellent that you will survive. Complications, including death, occur in 2 to 5 percent of these surgeries, depending on the surgeon and the cardiac team—and, of course, on your general physical condition. Older patients, or patients with other medical problems when they enter the operation, are more at risk of complications or even death.

So what I'm saying is that there is risk. We can do everything right during surgery and you can do everything right afterward, and that still doesn't guarantee that you won't have to have another surgery. In the majority of cases, the second operation isn't in any sense the fault of the patient. It just happens.

But there's an upside to this. You have a very good chance of getting through a second operation. Yeah, the odds in your favor have decreased, but they're still reasonably good. Another good thing is that most patients find the second experience easier than the first, partly because they know what to expect, partly because the procedures continue to improve. It's unusual to require a third operation—maybe 15 percent, or a little more, of those who go through a second must go through it one more time.

I wish I could sum all this up simply. I guess the closest I can get is that your best bet is to have good genes, not to smoke, to exercise and eat right, to control your blood pressure, and to never suffer heart disease in the first place.

Patient: At this point, I not only feel that I've gone through the procedure but that I could almost perform it on you!

Dr. Brenner: Good, that's the way I like it. We're partners in this, working toward the same end. I wouldn't want you to feel dehumanized by having to undergo this procedure. After all, it's the quality of your life we're talking about here. What we want is for you to have a second chance, to live the full and long life that we doctors like to think is everyone's birthright.

Patient: Thank you for that.

Chapter 5

RECOVERY AFTER BYPASS SURGERY

NORMA HENDON WOKE before dawn, her mind and heart racing so fast that she wondered if she'd slept at all. In only four hours, she thought. In only four hours, Gene, her husband of forty years, would have surgery. In only four hours he would undergo a procedure that could involve great pain for him, that might even cost him his life. In four hours his life would be in the hands of strangers—doctors and nurses whose incompetence or carelessness could cost Gene and her everything. And, if he survived, how would she care for him when he came home? And what if something went wrong while he was in her care?

Norma had asked the doctor these questions a thousand times, but now she remembered none of his reassuring answers. She remembered only one thing: in only four hours. . . . And then she remembered what had gotten her and her mother and her grandmother and generations of African women through tough times—unbending courage and strength and faith in God. So Norma fell to her knees and prayed that God would stay with her and Gene and their children through this frightening ordeal.

In a flurry of paper signing and presentation of insurance cards, Norma and Gene began to pass from their familiar world to a new one. But the new world, like the old, had its own human kindness. Norma was able to accompany Gene to his room and help him settle there. And the nurse who met them there, who obviously had seen a lot of these cases, looked them both in the eye and stated flatly that Gene would come out of this just fine. She inspired belief.

A few moments later, when Mrs. Hendon kissed her husband on the forehead and left him in the operating room, she needed all the faith and belief she could muster. For the long while that she sat alone in the surgical waiting room, she thought about the years they'd had together, the good times and the bad, and she felt overwhelmed with the generosity she'd known in the gift of love. Tears came, but she drew deeply on her strength and God's, and contained them. Gene needed her courage to feed his own. They were in this together. By the time her children arrived, she was composed and ready to calm and cheer them.

It was four long hours later when the cardiac surgeon walked in, a smile on his face, and told her that the surgery had gone perfectly, no complications, and Gene had come through fine. Yes, the operation had taken a little longer than he'd expected—there was a good deal of blockage, and he'd had to perform several bypasses.

"If you have any questions . . . ? Or maybe you just want to see Mr. Hendon?"

He took them to the intensive care unit (ICU), and when they walked into Gene's room, all Norma's fear returned. The room seemed full of bleeping monitors, and Gene lay there looking terribly helpless, tubes trailing from his mouth and nose, and a life support machine breathing for him. That was when Norma broke down for a moment, at the bedside, Gene's limp hand in hers. Though the nurses were there to comfort her and reassure her that this was all standard procedure and that Gene would soon be doing his own breathing, Norma didn't take the reassurance easily. She wished she'd been better prepared for this moment, but she knew that nothing could have prepared her. She'd never seen Gene stricken with anything worse than a cold. Now he was a person she had to stretch her imagination and heart to recognize, a man whose grasp on life depended on machines.

For Norma, a new and difficult time started, as Gene's long convalescence began. That healing process was as important to Gene's health and survival as the operation itself, and, if Norma entered this period in ignorance and fear, the convalescence would be a harsh ordeal for her and Gene as well.

Too many spouses, frightened as they are by the responsibilities of nursing, don't learn what's really needed to get through the convalescing period confidently and with at least a remnant of piece of mind. And, though we are sorry to say this, African Americans are sometimes less likely to ask the questions that can make the difference between being comfortable or not, or even between life and death.

There are many reasons this is true. In some cases, we have had bad experiences with doctors and nurses in the past, and meaningful communication was never established. Or it can simply be a matter of not knowing which questions to ask. Sometimes patients and their loved ones are muted by a kind of shyness: The doctors and nurses seem too busy to disturb. And anyway, they're the experts—they know what they're doing. We fear our questions will sound stupid to them. Maybe we will not ask the question right and they won't understand us.

Failure to ask questions can come from a kind of fatalism: The very trust in the Lord that can be a source of strength in medical crises can also be a source of weakness, if you put such complete trust in God and don't learn what is needed to convalesce well or to nurse a convalescent loved one. Remember what Bertha learned: In matters of coronary artery disease the Lord helps those who help themselves.

By understanding the process of recovery you will reduce the level of stress you'll feel.

But whatever the reasons (and they can be complicated, possibly stemming from bad, and sometimes racist, previous experience), it's our belief—indeed, it's the belief that drives this book—that we must understand the process of recovery lest we be paralyzed by paranoia and stress.

Once the period of surgery and hospitalization is over, a new team comes into play to help the patient—not the original team of doctors and nurses but a team of responsible family members and other professionals doing what they can to restore the patient to active and purposeful life.

Don't think that your questions and your desire to be useful will annoy the medical staff. Doctors and nurses respect and are grateful to family members who want to be part of the recovery effort. Doctors and nurses usually work hard, and a good family team makes their work a little easier. After all, no nursing can rival the nursing provided by those who are bound to the patient by love.

Of course, while the patient is still in the hospital, the family team should abide by the hospital's rules and schedules and regulations. That's easy enough. Norma learned much just by observing, and nurses were glad to tell her anything else she needed to know to make her efforts mesh with theirs. They appreciated her eager and willing cooperation and her active support of them and the doctors. No, they didn't ask her to help take blood samples, but they were glad for her help in getting Gene out of bed, in tidying around him, in helping with meals while he still needed help. Remember, recovery is a team effort between family and health care providers.

We know there are cases when, despite a family's best efforts, nurses or doctors don't take time to explain, or are simply rude. But when most doctors and nurses recognize that you and your family are caring, willing to listen and learn, willing to abide by the rules and eager to help, they will respond by providing the best care—which means, their all—to your loved one. After all, they too have feelings, and while they will carry out their responsibilities toward all patients, they're likely to reserve that extra best care for those whose families are ready to take a cheerful and active part in the recovery process.

THE FIRST STAGE OF RECOVERY

Recovery begins in the cardiac intensive care unit (also called a surgical ICU), where your loved one is taken after surgery. Though procedures vary from hospital to hospital, it is usual for the patient in the ICU to be under the care of at least one nurse, sometimes two. Their job is to monitor, with a machine that provides a constant reading of these functions, vital signs such as blood pressure, heart rate, oxygen blood levels, and other workings of the heart and lungs.

In the ICU the patient will usually be under the care of at least one nurse, sometimes two.

Because the patient was heavily sedated—in some cases, actually paralyzed—during surgery, some basic body functions have been weakened and have to be strengthened by still other machines and procedures until the patient recovers from anesthesia. The ventilator that helps him breathe will be gradually "weaned off" and then discontinued as he awakens. A catheter, or thin tube, placed in the bladder allows him to urinate spontaneously. And other tubes may be placed in the patient's chest to help drain excess blood from around the heart, where a buildup could interfere with the heartbeat and could require secondary surgery to correct. These tubes are usually removed one or two days after surgery.

The last such tube we must mention is the nasal gastric tube that, despite its name, is sometimes placed in the mouth instead of the nose. Its purpose is to keep the stomach empty, and though it looks uncomfortable, the anesthetized patient doesn't feel discomfort. Keeping the stomach empty helps to prevent food particles from entering the breathing pipe (trachea), with the possible result of pneumonia or other complications.

It's a dizzying and disturbing idea: Key functions of the body have been repressed or even stopped in order to carry out the surgery. And for a relatively brief while, these functions must still be carried out by machines. Without these machines and other technologies, this surgery could not be performed at all and the mortality rate would return to the higher levels that prevailed twenty years ago. So, though no one enjoys seeing a loved one rigged up with wires and tubes, the sight becomes a little easier when you understand why these are necessary.

There are other sights that disturbed Norma and may disturb you when you first see your loved one in the surgical ICU. When Norma walked into Gene's room in the ICU, she found that his hands were tied to the bed with straps. For a moment she was frightened and even angry. But the nurse explained that patients waking from anesthesia, four to six hours after the surgery is completed, are sometimes combative, which is a side effect of the anesthesia itself, or, in rare cases (two percent), this is due to strokes or other brain damage suffered as a result of surgery and a previously unstable condition. Left to their own devices, patients have been known to pull out chest tubes or other catheters. The reason is obvious: Patients are heavily sedated and aren't conscious of what's around them or even of their own behavior.

To prevent accidents from happening at this stage, nurses will sometimes use restraints on the patient's hands, until they're sure that the patient has awakened calmly. It's painful to see a loved one's hands tied to the bed, and especially painful to the uninformed. If someone is suspicious of the health system, as African Americans can sometimes be, the restraint may be interpreted as cruel or even racist. In general, at least, that's not the case. These restraints know no color barriers. Sometimes the patient can be talked into a calmer state; sometimes a light sedation is necessary. In any case, as soon as the patient becomes calm, the restraints are removed—and most patients awaken groggy but aware of where they are and able to talk to nurses and loved ones. That's how Gene was—somewhat uncomfortable and a little goofy, but glad to see Norma, and glad that he had come through the surgery.

After heart surgery, patients often are swollen. Gene was, all over, and it frightened Norma to see him that way. But instead of panicking, she asked the nurse about it and learned that the swelling was because of the transfusions of blood and other fluids Gene had received and retained while on the bypass machine. It would vanish, the nurse explained, within 24 to 48 hours after surgery. Norma was also bothered to see Gene wrapped in a warming blanket, despite the normal temperature of the room. She learned that warming is necessary because surgery is often performed in a very cold room in order to preserve the heart, and afterward the patient must recover the warmth he lost.

After heart surgery, patients often are swollen – it's normal.

Again, we don't claim that because you understand the reason for all these devices and procedures you won't be upset to see your loved one engulfed in them. But knowing why they are necessary may make their impact a little easier to take. By the end of the surgery day, Norma felt exhausted, but she was also relieved. Gene was alive, he was recovering, and she knew that a new phase of their lives was beginning. It might be difficult, perhaps, but certainly not all bad. They had each other, and if they could adjust to Gene's new status as a postsurgical coronary artery surgery patient, they had years of happiness to look forward to.

THE SECOND STAGE OF RECOVERY

The second stage of the surgical recovery cycle, known as postoperative day one, or, simply, POD 1, can be the beginning of a new happiness, because it's the day when the patient begins to take steps toward a normal life. To be sure, on POD 1, and for several days afterward, the patient's EKG, heart rhythm, and blood pressure will continue to be monitored. This is necessary because the heart that has undergone bypass surgery can still be irritable until it heals. The EKG and other monitors usually catch such problems at once so that they can be treated before they become serious.

But the very good news is that chest tubes, bladder and nasal catheters are now removed. At this point, family members or other loved ones can be very helpful. Norma was glad to be able to assist Gene in drinking. Because his blood pressure and other vital signs were stable, he was put on a liquid diet of water, juices, or broth once the breathing tube was removed. With Norma's assistance, Gene also enjoyed a sponge bath—not a shower, because the incisions heal fastest if they are kept dry for the first five to seven days after surgery.

Norma was able to help Gene sit up and to remind him to breathe and cough. This may sound silly, but Gene needed reminders. He'd had a deep incision through the breast bone and flesh, and despite medication, that incision hurt. So the nurses, and Norma, helped him to sit up in bed and dangle his legs, and, later, to sit up in a chair. Before going to sleep that night, Gene was walking around the ICU with a little help from Norma and the nurse.

Some patients may feel that it is asking too much to make them sit up or even walk around only ten hours after heart surgery, but the vast majority (98 percent) are able to do this and will be encouraged to. Such activity, along with breathing exercises, is essential to recovery. Patients who do best at respiratory treatments, with the help of family, nurses, and respiratory therapists, will recuperate more strongly and will be allowed to leave the hospital earlier than those who don't.

Patients are encouraged to sit up or even walk around only ten hours after heart surgery. The vast majority (98%) are able to do this.

If the patient has been a smoker, the breathing problem is more complicated and there is more danger of respiratory problems such as a collapsed lung or bronchitis, or the buildup of mucus secretions that can lead to pneumonia. So for smokers, breathing treatments are especially needed.

Usually, for patients recovering from heart surgery, respiratory treatments occur every four hours around the clock, and it's absolutely essential that they be carried out with the patient's full cooperation. Doctors often use a device called an incentive spirometry, which helps the lungs to expand more fully. The device is held to the patient's mouth while the patient takes a deep breath, drawing air into the lungs to expand them and sometimes to help clear secretions that accumulate during the operation while the patient is on the bypass machine.

Family members should express their willingness to assist the nurses in the various therapies that occur on POD1. Often, only you will be able to say the right encouraging word, and you may be able to assist physically as well. But remember that your encouraging should be gentle, supportive, and positive, not critical. If you can sympathize with your loved one's discomfort and pain, and at the same time lend him or her your courage and love, you will become an essential part of the recuperation process.

THE THIRD STAGE OF RECOVERY

POD2 is an extension and acceleration of POD1. The patient's breathing exercises are increased. The patient is asked to sit up in a chair three or four times a day and to walk in the ICU or in the step-down unit. Transfer to a step-down unit is another measure of recovery. Here, the patient is still monitored, but less intensively than in the ICU. Although transfer to this unit is a clear sign that the patient is on the way to recovery, the patient, with the help of you and the nurses, must continue to work.

Remember that recovery from major surgery is not like recovery from a cold. It requires serious work from the patient at a time when he is barely able to perform it. The core work, as before, is deep breathing and walking. Because it is common for a patient to feel worse on the second day than on the first, your kind words to the loved one, your ability to see the big picture and to convey it to him, can make a world of difference. Remind him that he is getting better even though he may not be feeling better. You'll only be telling him the truth.

Along with encouragement, there are certain restraints to be placed on the patient's activity. For instance, he should never walk without help from you or from a nurse. Patients like Gene who underwent conventional bypass surgery, involving splitting the breast bone, are instructed not to lift anything heavier than 8 to 10 pounds. The danger is that the breast bone can split open again. But that rarely occurs if the patient follows directions carefully.

THE FOURTH STAGE OF RECOVERY

On days three and four, the patient is expected to walk farther and to perform the breathing exercises more aggressively. Gene's appetite was still poor, but the nurse assured Norma it would improve over time. Because Gene wasn't yet having bowel movements, he felt uncomfortable. When he complained about this to Norma, she talked to the nurse and a laxative solved the problem. On the third day, in Gene's case—or sometimes on day four—chest x-rays and lab work, including a red blood cell count along with electrolytes, were done. That those tests were ordered, the nurse explained, was a good sign: They were part of the preparation for Gene's going home, as he did on day four. Most patients leave the hospital between days three and five.

Most patients leave the hospital after three to five days.

Naturally, Norma felt some anxiety about Gene's discharge, since responsibility for his well-being shifted from the medical staff to her. Now, more than ever, it was important for her to understand Gene's capacities as well as his incapacities. She would become the medical staff, the dietitian, and to some extent the rehabilitation therapist. We don't pretend that these are easy responsibilities. But we can say confidently that the more you know in advance about what to expect, the better nurse you will be.

This next stage begins while still at the hospital. Before Gene was discharged, Norma talked with a dietitian about a proper heart-healthy diet. (And we'll talk to you about this later in the book.) Norma was also careful, as the doctor had suggested, to have Gene scheduled for cardiac rehabilitation. In a broad sense, this is simply a routine that a person who has undergone heart surgery must follow from the day he is discharged through the rest of his life. It involves exercising, eating well, and, obviously, discontinuing smoking and controlling blood pressure. It should all begin at once, as soon as the patient has had a chance to adjust to being home.

It is essential that you enter a cardiac rehabilitation program, and that you be sure to take daily walks.

Gene and Norma celebrated their return by taking a walk together around the house, and, since Gene had the energy, by walking around the block, accepting the good wishes of several neighbors. The next day, since the weather was bad, they went to the shopping mall, where Gene walked for quite a while, taking pleasure in the people, especially the children. On other days, they walked in a neighborhood park. Though Gene was still weak, the joy of returning to familiar spots and breathing clean air was energizing.

Much of the responsibility for recovery fell on Gene himself, but Norma's encouragement and support, her gentle reminders, helped him establish the healthy routines he needed—in some cases, replacing the unhealthy ones that led to surgery in the first place.

While the most important elements of cardiac rehabilitation occur at home, we strongly encourage you, as the patient, to join a structured rehabilitation program for at least a month or two after surgery. If the doctor hasn't already scheduled you for such a program before you leave the hospital, remind him or her. The program ensures that you will continue to be monitored so that your doctor can evaluate how well you are doing and can identify potential problems that might arise.

We don't consider it necessary that, as part of the rehabilitation, you buy an exercise bicycle or other expensive equipment. It is essential that you enter a cardiac rehabilitation program and that you take daily walks.

Remember that recovery is a process: It does not occur in the wink of an eye. In some ways, it is like being born again—that is, you must regain the strength and agility that you always took for granted. You can walk, even climb stairs. But you must not at first try to use your strength as before. Lifting can be especially dangerous, because it can open the incision itself or split the breast bone. Until the doctor is satisfied that these wounds are satisfactorily healed, you should not lift anything over 8 or 10 pounds.

Remember: recovery is a process, it does not occur in the wink of an eye.

If your loved one has had surgery, one of the jobs you can perform at this stage is to keep an eye on the wounds, changing the dressing as instructed by the doctor, and regularly examining the wounds—the one in the chest and the one in the leg where the vein was removed—to ensure that they're healing properly.

If you see signs that the wound isn't healing properly, inform the doctor or nurse at once. For that matter, if you have any doubts, arrange for a visit or simply call the doctor. A serious complication that can occur after open heart surgery is an infection, either in the chest or the leg. It's urgent that this problem be reported so that antibiotics can be administered as soon as possible. In such cases, the patient should not bathe or use any ointment other than those the doctor has prescribed.

The doctor will probably ask that the patient not drive a car for the first several weeks, because of the possibility of colliding with the steering wheel and hitting the breast bone if an accident were to occur. The doctor will also ask the patient not to engage in sexual relations for four to six weeks. Obviously, neither the excitement nor the physical exertion is appropriate for a recovering heart patient.

If there is any recurrence of the symptoms suffered before the surgery—shortness of breath, chest pressure, rapid heart rate, sweating at night, excessive swelling, or just plain not feeling right—call the doctor at once. If you can't reach the doctor, or even if the doctor takes the symptoms less seriously than you do, go to the emergency room. It's best to follow your gut instincts, even if that means going against your doctor's assurance. A trip to the emergency room will cost you little and could save your loved one's life.

THE RECOVERING PATIENT'S RESPONSIBILITIES

Yes, convalescence has its dangers, just as the operation did. It's our job to tell you about them, and it's your job to do what you can to avoid them, or, if they appear, to recognize and do something about them as soon as possible. But there is also something wonderful about returning to the activities of a normal life. And there are many paths open to the patient, as long as he or she is patient.

The worst thing a patient can do is to sit like a vegetable while people wait on him hand and foot. Here are some of the things the patient can and should do:

- Clean and bathe himself or herself.
- Cook and light cleaning.
- Do light chores such as setting the table, washing dishes, and picking up clothing.

Even if the patient did not ordinarily do such things in the past, let him start now. Such chores are good for him physically and are good for household morale. Besides, there's nothing better for a patient than to feel useful again.

People who were active or athletic before the operation—for example, Bigger in chapter three—may want to return too quickly to their old sports or workouts. Obviously, that's to be avoided. The rule is: Take it slow but take it. For the first month, no lifting of anything over 8 to 10 pounds, no strenuous exertion, no driving, and no sexual activity. If your doctor's own protocol is a little different from ours, by all means, follow it. But whatever the plan, what it requires from the recuperating person is patience, perseverance, and faith that if you take it slow you will soon be enjoying your life again as much—or more—than you ever did.

RECOVERY AND RENEWAL

Norma and Gene discovered that recovery is a family affair. When Gene was distracted—and, given the ordeal he'd been through and the discomfort he still felt, he sometimes was—Norma helped by reminding him to take his medications as scheduled. She also made a point of redefining home cooking. In the past, too many of their favorite dishes were loaded with fat and cholesterol, and, because they were both busy, the family diet sometimes relied too heavily on fast foods, as it commonly does in American families today, and especially in African American ones. Norma took it upon herself to change that, and, to her surprise and delight, Gene himself got interested in cooking. They both discovered that tasty African American cooking can be lean cuisine without sacrificing flavor, as you'll see later in this book.

Recovery is a family affair. Shedding bad habits together and cultivating good ones will give the entire family a sense of renewal.

Gene didn't smoke, but if he had, it wouldn't be enough for him to stop. Other members of the household would have to—or at least should—stop also. It does little good for the patient to stop smoking only to be subjected to second-hand smoke, which studies show contributes not only to coronary artery disease but to cancer as well. Recuperation can be a family affair, a team effort. Shedding bad habits together and cultivating good ones will give the entire family a sense of renewal. And while you are eliminating risk factors and practicing rehabilitation together, the whole household may go through the experience of healing with the patient.

Rehabilitation is a kind of renewal. Many patients find that as difficult as the recovery period may be, it carries with it a kind of hidden gift. If life has become more fragile than it seemed before, it has also become more precious. Convalescence is a kind of second gift of life, a second helping. Some patients find that it is oddly better than the first, since it presents, inescapably, the great richness of simple things. Just as the recovering patient may find that, instead of heavy second helpings of turkey and dressing and gravy, he has become content with more parsnips and turnips, so he may find that in other areas of life, not the old ambitions and desires and excitements drive him, but something quieter and more true.

A SHORT QUIZ

How well have you learned your lessons? Here's a little quiz.

1. Once you've checked into the hospital with your loved one, (a) you won't see him again until after the operation, (b) you'll be able to accompany him to his room and remain with him until it's time for him to be taken to surgery, (c) you'll be able to accompany him to surgery, or (d) you won't see him again until he is out of the intensive care unit.

2. When you first see your loved one after the operation, he may (a) be hooked up to machines, (b) have tubes in his mouth or nose, as well as in his arms, (c) look swollen, or (d) all of these.

3. Asking questions of the doctors or nurses after the operation is likely to (a) annoy them, (b) make them suspect that you're stupid, (c) give them the opportunity to show off, or (d) gain their respect and help assure you that your loved one will enjoy their extra best efforts.

4. When your loved one wakes up from anesthesia, (a) there's nothing you can do for him, (b) you can assist him in sitting up and doing his breathing exercises,

(c) you can get him ready to go home, or (d) you can expect him to be pretty much as usual.

5. If you find your loved one's hands tied with sheets to the bed, you should (a) complain to a nurse, (b) get a lawyer, (c) untie them, or (d) know that this is to control his movements until he's awakened and calm.

6. Usually, on the day after the operation the patient will (a) be free of all monitors and tubes, (b) still be linked to monitors, (c) still be connected to chest and nasal tubes, or (d) be ready to go home.

7. Patients recovering from heart surgery should be able to walk (a) only after a week, (b) within an hour after awakening, (c) within 6 to 10 hours of awakening, or (d) only after a month.

8. Respiratory treatments are needed (a) to help keep the lungs clear of secretions that may accumulate there, (b) because the patient may not breathe as well due to pain, (c) because they give the patient something to do, or (d) both a and b.

9. Once they are home, patients (a) can resume all their normal physical activities, (b) should be allowed to drive as soon as they feel like it, (c) should begin serious weight training, or (d) should not lift weights of more than 8 to 10 pounds.

10. If the patient has been a smoker, (a) he should be allowed to continue smoking, (b) he shouldn't smoke, but it's all right if other members of the family do, (c) he should be rationed to two or three cigarettes a day, or (d) both the patient and other household members should give up smoking at once.

11. In order to rehabilitate the patient, you should (a) buy an exercise bicycle or other aerobic exercise machine, (b) get him to join a gym, (c) hire a physical therapist, or (d) be sure that he walks regularly and carries out breathing exercises.

The answers, as we probably don't have to tell you, are 1b, 2d, 3d, 4b, 5d, 6b, 7c, 8d, 9d, 10d, 11d.

Chapter 6

HAVING A HEART ATTACK AND SURVIVING

EACH YEAR THERE ARE over a million new or recurrent heart attack cases in the United States. Death results in about a third of these cases. The aim of this chapter is to ensure that, should you suffer a heart attack, you survive it. You have a good chance if you live through the first hour and get immediate and appropriate treatment. So, to a degree, at least, surviving is in your hands and the hands of your loved ones.

Each year there are over 1,000,000 new or recurrent heart attack cases in this country.

People who suffer heart attacks all too often try to deny what is happening to them: "I am too young!" "No, this is something that happens to other people!" "I'm just panicked!" "I shouldn't have eaten that second chili dog!" Unfortunately, heart attack doesn't leave much time for denial. Doctors refer to the first hour of a heart attack as the "golden hour" because that's the optimal time for you to get to the hospital and, where appropriate, be treated with either the clot-busting medications, angioplasty, stenting, or bypass surgery that may save your life.

The clot-busters, or thrombolytics, by breaking up the clots in your arteries, help restore the blood flow to the heart and thus decrease the damage. As you know, a heart attack occurs because blockages prevent blood from getting to the heart. During that period of blood starvation, the heart weakens and can die. Once it dies, it cannot be restored. Thrombolytics work within one to six hours from the beginning of the heart attack, and the later the medications are administered, the less likely they will do any good. After 6 hours, the part of the heart suffering the heart attacks dies permanently.

Perhaps nothing we say in this book is of greater potential importance to you than the following:

- If you think you are suffering a heart attack, take two aspirins, crushed, and call 911.
- Don't call your doctor or the local hospital—just call 911.
- Don't attempt to drive yourself and don't let your loved ones drive. Wait for the ambulance to come. That way you will get treated faster during the early stages of the heart attack and have a better chance at survival.
- If the attack is happening to someone else, call 911. There's no time for denial or for lengthy discussion. Life is hanging on a thread.

The higher mortality rates from heart attacks experienced by African Americans suggest a stronger tendency toward denial in these matters. Sometimes that denial results from a failure to associate the symptoms with their serious cause, and to attribute them instead to a secondary cause such as indigestion. Sometimes, bad experience with the medical system makes you mistrust it. And sometimes denial is caused by unfamiliarity with the emergency medical system or fear of embarrassment that you might be wrong if the symptoms turn out to have a less serious cause.

If you think you are suffering a heart attack, take two aspirins, crushed, and call 911.

Certainly that happens, and we can all be glad for it. In fact, 85 percent of the patients who go to the emergency room believing they are having a heart attack are not. Don't be embarrassed. If you believe that you or a loved one is suffering the symptoms we describe in this chapter, call 911. If you are proven wrong, rejoice to be in the majority. Let a doctor decide the seriousness of the episode.

Panic disorder is especially likely to be mistaken for a heart attack. Panic disorders are real, and the symptoms can include chest pressure or pain, a racing heart, shortness of breath, lightheadedness, chills or flushes, numbness of the arms, and trembling of the fingers—in short, symptoms that closely resemble the more serious symptoms of a heart attack.

Don't try to make this difficult distinction yourself. Only the emergency room doctor should do that. We can say that the symptoms of a panic attack don't last long and won't take your life. In the end, the attack is harmless, however unpleasant. Once you have calmed down, you're as good as new. In the case of a heart attack, of course, the symptoms persist.

Again, these matters aren't the stuff of guessing games. If you must err, err on the side of prudence. If you're really suffering a heart attack, the longer you wait, the more likelihood of serious damage or the more likelihood you will die. Remember, one hour is the optimal time period, the "golden hour." During the first six hours the thrombolytics can help you. During that same period, your doctor may use angioplasty, stenting, or bypass surgery in an effort to restore blood to your heart. After that period, permanent damage is likely to have occurred and your chance of long-term survival is dramatically shortened.

THE WARNING SIGNS OF A HEART ATTACK

The leading symptoms of a heart attack include:

- A sensation of pressure in the center of the chest. This may be experienced as an uncomfortable fullness, or a squeezing pain, or a great weight, like a vice, or an elephant sitting on your chest. This discomfort is sometimes accompanied by light-headedness, fainting, sweating, nausea, or shortness of breath. If these symptoms last more than a few minutes, you may be experiencing a heart attack.
- Pain spreading to the shoulders, neck, or arms. It may also affect the jaw and the eyes. Once again, if it lasts more than a few minutes you must take it as a symptom.

If you are already on a prescription of nitroglycerin and these sensations don't vanish after you take the medication, you must treat them as symptoms. Not all these symptoms occur in every attack. And they may go away and return again. But if they persist, get help fast.

WHEN DO HEART ATTACKS USUALLY OCCUR?

Heart attacks often occur upon waking in the morning when the heart rouses from its restful state. Ordinarily this is a process it takes in stride, and an increased blood flow follows the awakened demands of the heart. But if there is an underlying problem, the inability of the arteries to deliver the needed blood can trigger an attack.

Heart attacks often occur when we wake up in the morning and the heart rouses from its restful state.

Times of heavy exertion can also bring on an attack. We've all heard stories of people struck down while shoveling snow, lifting a hay bale, or doing something else that exerts them to the utmost.

Emotional extremes, just like physical ones, can cause an attack. Excesses of joy, even excesses of grief or rage, can set the process in motion. Oddly, in the case of extreme emotions, heart attacks sometimes occur two hours after the outburst. The extreme emotion, whether good or bad, brings about an increase in adrenaline (i.e., epinephrine), which causes the heart rate and blood pressure to increase and also causes the blood to clot more easily. As this process runs its course, a heart attack can ensue.

All these potential causes are even more of a risk to a person who has already suffered a heart attack. As we'll see later in this chapter, it isn't as if such survivors must live as if they're walking on eggshells. They simply must do what they can to avoid physical and emotional extremes.

WHAT YOU CAN DO IN THE CASE OF A HEART ATTACK

You know the symptoms: chest pain or prolonged pressure, pain spreading to the shoulders, neck, or arms, perhaps to the jaw and eyes. The first problem you face when confronted with these symptoms in yourself or someone close to you is to stay calm. If the patient gets agitated, he or she only complicates the problem by increasing the heart rate and the blood pressure.

In the event of a heart attack Keep Calm!

Obviously, it's not easy to remain calm when you sense that you or your loved one may die. We don't pretend that we have a magic prescription for keeping calm under such circumstances. But we do believe that the better you know what to do, the more likely you are to switch into an action mode, which is one way of overriding panic.

If you are the one who is having the attack, call 911 and ask for an ambulance, or have someone else do it for you. If you are caring for someone suffering the attack, make the call immediately. Only if there is well-founded doubt about the availability of an ambulance should you take the patient to the hospital yourself.

If you are the victim, don't try to drive yourself. And don't try to walk to the hospital. You need help. Speed is absolutely of the essence here. Remember, your aim is to get to the hospital before an hour passes. If you are the caregiver in such a situation, expect denial on the part of the victim, and find a way to overcome his or her objection. The victim may try to convince you that what he or she is suffering is unimportant and will pass in a moment. He won't want to spoil his evening, or yours. He won't want to bother you. Fear itself may make him think that going to the hospital is a way of conceding that he's close to death, and he may do everything he can to avoid going. You must rely on your knowledge that chest pain or unusual pressure is a heart attack until proven otherwise. Don't take no for an answer—get the victim to the hospital.

If you are the caregiver of a patient suffering a heart attack, expect denial on the part of the victim, and find a way to overcome their objection.

If the victim has suffered actual cardiac arrest and has fallen over, check for a pulse by placing your hands along the victim's neck or your index and middle fingers on the wrist. If you feel no pulse, you need to start CPR—cardio pulmonary resuscitation. Everyone who lives with a person with heart problems or in a family in which heart attacks have been common should learn this simple technique. Too many people die because no one around them knows CPR. So wisdom suggests that, long before you need to use the procedure, you should call your local hospital or Red Cross and sign up for a free class. Don't let a loved one die because you didn't have the necessary skills when they were needed.

If the victim has not suffered cardiac arrest and is conscious and on her feet, your first job is to calm her and lay her down, placing a pillow underneath her knees. Don't let her try to walk or do anything that places an unnecessary strain on the heart.

Loosen all tight clothing and open a window to provide fresh air. If the person has already been diagnosed as having heart disease and has been prescribed nitroglycerin, administer it to relieve the chest discomfort. The American Heart Association also suggests that two or three aspirin, preferably crushed and dissolved in water, should be administered at this point. As an anticoagulant, aspirin can help slow down the heart attack and reduce damage. Do not give the victim anything else to eat or drink, because that could cause breathing problems.

Let's review your job if you are the witness of a heart attack:

1. Stay cool and calm and try to calm the victim.
2. Make the victim as comfortable as possible.
3. Administer nitroglycerin if available and/or two or three crushed or dissolved aspirins.
4. Call the 911 operator, who will direct an ambulance to your home. Don't waste time calling other numbers.
5. If, after calling 911, there's well-founded uncertainty about getting an ambulance, take the patient to the hospital yourself, doing what you can to minimize physical or emotional strain on him or her.

EMERGENCY CARE AT THE HOSPITAL

The first thing the emergency medical crew will do once they've determined you're experiencing a heart attack is administer agents that will help break up the clotting and thus allow more blood to flow to the heart. This will limit the damage to the heart. Then you will be admitted to the cardiac care unit (CCU), where you will be placed on a monitor that gives a constant EKG (electrocardiogram) reading. The purpose is to identify dangerous arrhythmias that sometimes occur after a heart attack. If they are detected, they can often be corrected. The EKG also helps detect whether the heart is ischemic—that is, suffering from decreased blood flow. While all this is going on, the medical staff will do lab tests that will tell them definitively whether you've had a heart attack.

Remember that most deaths from heart attacks occur within the first hour from the time the symptoms appear. If you make it through that time period, your chances of survival are good. And if you are alive one month after a life-threatening attack, you have a 70 to 80 percent chance of living the next five years. Many people, of course, survive a good deal longer than that.

RECUPERATION

Ordinarily, for at least the first twelve hours in the CCU, you'll be kept in bed. After that, you'll be encouraged to move around to decrease the risk of blood clots. (Each hospital has its own procedures, but that's the usual course.) Your cardiologist may wish to perform a cardiac catheterization to determine the extent of your coronary artery disease.

Patients in CCU may experience serious confusion and disorientation, sometimes hallucinations. Added to the fear of having experienced a heart attack, these states can be very disturbing. All we can give you here in the way of comfort is reassurance that these situations are common. They're caused by the decreased flow of blood to the brain, which results in changes to thought patterns.

If you are suffering these symptoms, it may not be easy to control them. If your agitation is severe, your nurse will help you by administering either Valium or morphine sulfate—drugs that will help relieve anxiety or pain. Such states must be controlled because, as you know, stress is bad for your heart. Not only does it mean increased heart rate and blood pressure but it also makes blood more sticky and likely to clot—a condition that can cause further heart attacks.

You'll find ways to pass the time during your period in CCU. Reading, listening to music, watching TV (stay clear of programs full of agitation), talking to others—all these things will help you return to normal life. Prayer can help, as can any positive act on your part. Brooding is best avoided.

We don't pretend that everyone finds this period of recovery easy. For some, especially those who suffered from depression before the attack, depression may accompany the anxiety or follow it. It comes with a message of sadness and powerlessness, a lack of energy and motivation. You may find that your appetites are diminished, whether for food or sex. The activities that once made you happy may offer nothing to you now. If all this gets bad enough, thoughts of suicide may occur. Some 30 percent of those who have had severe heart trouble, like heart attacks, suffer from depression.

Depression can have a negative impact on your recovery. As a predictor that you will have further heart problems, it's potentially as bad as high cholesterol or even smoking. That's why you will need to lean on others during this time. If you are lucky, you'll have family and friends to give you the support and encouragement you need. If not, nurses will prove important human contact. Further, nurses can arrange visits by a social worker or minister who knows how to give comfort and support. Remember that as you recover you are at an important turning point. You've survived and you've been given the opportunity to change your life and improve it. Many others have turned this calamity into the beginning of a new and better life, and you can too.

REHABILITATION AFTER CCU

After you've been transferred from CCU to a regular ward, you'll eventually enter a cardiac rehabilitation program. The program will teach you how to reduce stress and it will recommend an exercise program appropriate to your condition. It will also encourage you to share your experiences with others in the same boat so that your individual work toward recovery can be strengthened by the experiences of the group. Finally, the program will regularly monitor your heart after exercise in order to evaluate how effective the surgical or medical treatment has been.

Cardiac rehabilitation will go on for the rest of your life.

Don't think of cardiac rehabilitation as something that goes on only until you are released from the hospital. In fact, it will go on all your life. We think this should be happy news. It means that for the rest of your life you will be giving your body the attention it needs and you will be giving your emotional life the same active attention. Admittedly, for those who hadn't been taking care of these matters before the heart attack, the shift requires new resolution. But you will be working with the advantage of the severe warning you've been given by your heart. What greater cause for thanksgiving than this grand second chance?

The aims of cardiac rehabilitation, besides the crucial aim of strengthening your heart to get you through the effects of the first attack and to reduce the chance of a second one, are:

- To decrease your cholesterol level
- To reverse or slow down coronary disease
- To improve your energy level
- To teach you to exercise
- To help you control stress and depression
- To move you toward a fresh and healthier outlook on life

Renewal and rehabilitation can be among the supreme human experiences.

Renewal and rehabilitation can be among the supreme human experiences, in their own way like experiencing conversion, or learning faith in the Lord. Your work in cardiac rehabilitation involves more than exercise of the heart and body, though there will be plenty of that. It also means changes in your diet, in your way of dealing with stress, and in your general outlook on yourself and others. For some, it may mean coming to grips with emotional and social problems that have haunted them for years. Obviously, there is much strength and spirit in such work.

WHAT THE FAMILY CAN DO

Although we've naturally been focusing on the problems of the patient, family members also face special problems when someone close to them has had a heart attack. For many African Americans, these problems can be made worse by past experiences of poor medical treatment and racism, perhaps even at the hands of doctors or other providers. Naturally, African American families will want their loved one to receive the best care and not second-class treatment.

Rather than suffer such fears silently, it's better to voice them. Yes, it's possible to do so, tactfully but frankly. Better yet, because you've been forearmed with knowledge, you know what treatment to expect. If your loved one isn't getting it, ask why. Recognize that there may be legitimate explanations. Not all hospital procedures are the same. But it is reasonable to make sure that the treatment is the best possible, and the doctors or nurses should recognize the legitimacy of your concern. By practicing politeness and persistence, you can ensure that they will give you their best.

There's another problem that the family member may face. When you see a close relative helpless, you may have a selfish thought: How can this person keep up with his or her share of responsibility? That responsibility can take a thousand forms—child care, income for food and rent, household duties, companionship, and emotional support.

Worse, if the loved one has suffered permanent damage and is disabled either permanently or for what's likely to be a long period, you may have to think about nursing care, with all the costs and trouble that involves. Such a responsibility can be devastating when, added to it, there is loss of the patient's income. And even in cases where no income is lost, nursing is expensive and can put great strains on the budget.

The impact of these matters on the survivor can result in guilt and depression, which are bad for the survivor's heart. In some cases, where you may have had a fight with the loved one before the attack, or where you feel that you ignored signs and symptoms you should have been mindful of, you can also feel guilty. Or you may simply feel angry at the new responsibilities placed on you and the loss of companionship that has resulted.

Sometimes that tumult of emotions leads to outbursts against the very medical staff that is caring for your loved one. Keep that possibility in mind and try to sort out your feelings. Otherwise, you may find yourself taking them out on people who are often doing their best. If you scold them needlessly, or blow up at them, you can set in motion a kind of self-fulfilling prophecy, and you may find that your loved one actually begins to get less careful attention. Remember that medical people have feelings too.

All we can say to help you here is that in most cases medical staff are doing the work they love and are usually doing it to the best of their ability. Most of them took on the work because they wished to be useful to others. For your part, take advantage of the extended family. Air your concerns with family members who aren't as deeply emotionally involved as you are. They may help you to find solutions for the burdens you may suddenly face. And they may give you better perspective on the actions of the medical staff. Your minister or social worker can also be useful at this stage, both in helping you find solutions and helping you gain perspective.

Again, it will help you too to know all you can about the medical situation. Write your questions on a piece of paper and leave room for the answers. At a teaching hospital, you may find yourself putting the questions to a resident or intern or nurse. In most cases, they will know their stuff and tell you what you need to know. If you're not satisfied, you have the right to talk to the doctor. Simply ask the intern or nurse to make an appointment for you.

Here are a few questions you may wish to ask:

- Why did this happen?
- Exactly what did happen and how extensive and serious is the heart damage?
- What immediate complications could occur and what long-range ones?
- What treatment is the loved one getting, and is there anything in that treatment that departs from the standard?
- What reading material does the doctor have available that would help you learn more about coronary artery disease and heart attacks?

Such knowledge will help you in caring for and encouraging your loved one. Finally, by asking questions, you'll gain the respect of the medical staff. Doctors and nurses respond to people who, whether or not they have formal education, take the trouble to educate themselves about the medical problem they face. And, we must say, they will be all the more likely to ensure that your loved one gets the best possible care. It's simply human nature that we reserve our best for those we feel a personal human connection with. At the same time, you're preparing yourself to be a more effective caregiver.

Doctors and nurses respond to people who, whether or not they have formal education, take the trouble to educate themselves about the medical problem they face.

SEX AFTER A HEART ATTACK

You may be embarrassed to ask the doctor or nurse about sex, but it's an important part of most of our lives, and the survivor of a heart attack, along with the person with whom he or she shared a bed, must know what can be done and what can't after a heart attack.

A person who has had a heart attack, stroke, or coronary artery bypass grafting will, for some time afterward, have a decreased sexual appetite and will certainly feel less sexy. If you keep yourself reasonably active physically after a heart attack, it is less likely that resuming sex will be a problem. Exercise at least two or three times a week.

There are circumstances that increase the risk of suffering a second heart attack during or after sexual activity. You may find it odd that extramarital affairs pose a special danger. Guilt and fear of getting caught increase stress, and you know that's bad for the heart. Further, the extramarital lover is more likely to be trying to demonstrate sexual prowess and overexert him- or herself. A silly but common and potentially serious problem is that, under such circumstances, the heart attack survivor who feels pain or chest pressure during sex may be embarrassed to take nitroglycerin. Finally, extramarital sex may be more often accompanied by other indulgences—in alcohol, tobacco, or even illicit drugs.

For these reasons, we don't recommend that you make extramarital sex part of your cardiac rehabilitation program. As to marital sex, talk to your doctor about when you can resume sexual activity. If you find it easier, you can talk to him or her over the phone. Most doctors will respond readily to such questions. But get answers that are personal and specific to your case.

YOUR NEW LIFE

A brush with death is a powerful and wonderful motivator. So is the threat of a second brush. That's why so many people have found their heart attack a strong reason to reshape their lives. We hope that you'll be one of them, so here are some tips for getting started.

You'll want to avail yourself, through your doctor, of the best, most current medical information. Medicine is always changing and you need to be kept up-to-date.

Along with information, you'll need vision. By this we mean simply that, once you've committed yourself to changing your life, you'll want literally to visualize the benefits that will come to you as a result. Thus, before you exercise, picture yourself feeling healthier and looking better and more fit. Call on those images frequently to strengthen your choice of a new, healthier life.

Eat well and in moderation, and exercise regularly—ideally, three times a week. Each day do something, no matter how small, to change yourself for the better. By building confidence in small changes, you will strengthen your resolve in the big ones.

Take time each day to meditate, pray, or simply clarify your values. Type A personalities, people on the fast track, determined to excel at whatever they're doing, often get out of the habit of stopping to rest, or of getting in touch with their deeper feelings. Those omissions helped get them to the CCU in the first place. Now they must be corrected.

Take time each day, a regular time, to meditate, pray, or simply clarify your values.

Stress and steadily living on the run is bad for the healthy. But they're especially bad for the person who has already been struck down by a heart that wasn't getting the right kind of attention and care. Now, as you return to normal life, you will be subjected once again to all the pressure and stress that life brings to all of us. Choose your company carefully. Instead of long lunches with hyped-up friends or colleagues who are drinking and smoking, cultivate friends who are health conscious and understand the benefits of calm and emotional balance.

Fear may motivate you at first, but as you work to make yourself new, you'll find that the powerful sense of renewal will soon displace that fear.

Big changes require planning, sustained purpose, care for the details, and an eye on the benefits that the changes are designed to bring. Fear may motivate you at first, but as you work to make yourself new, you'll find that the powerful sense of renewal will soon displace that fear. We've said it before and we'll say it again: Millions have found their second lives better than their first. You can too, with goodwill, patience, and a little help from your friends and loved ones. And faith in something bigger than yourself can make all the difference in the world.

Chapter 7

CONGESTIVE HEART FAILURE

When Sara Williams woke at 6 A.M., as she always did, she heard her two sons breathing and mumbling in their sleep. Drew, the younger, was still sleeping in the room he'd had when he was a boy. Now he was thirty but hadn't left home. He'd held some fly-by-night jobs, and once or twice taken an apartment of his own for a few months, but he always came back. He needed to find himself, he'd tell his mother, and that's what she'd tell her friends, a little embarrassed. "He's a good boy," she'd say, "smart and able. Once he decides what he wants to do, he does just fine."

Bryan, who slept on the sofa, was a harder case, from Sara's point of view. He worked steadily, managing a furniture store, but when he got divorced six months ago he ended up on her doorstep. "Divorce is like sickness, Ma," he told her. "I just have to have time to get over it and decide where I want to live."

Sara didn't get much help from her boys. Once in a while she thought they ought to be looking after her by now, but mostly she just did what she had to do. The boys brought in some money, and she cooked and kept house.

Her husband Will had died two years ago. Once or twice she'd thought how nice it would be to marry again, to have the kind of warm and joking companionship she'd had with Will. But, no, she said to herself, that would be disrespectful to him, disrespectful to her family. Once she'd decided that, she couldn't see much reason for taking care of herself as she had when Will was around. She'd put on a few pounds, she didn't have the energy she used to have, and her breathing wasn't as easy as she'd like it to be. But when it bothered her, as now, when she tried to sleep or rest in bed, she'd just put another pillow behind her and that gave her a little relief.

In fact, Sara was only sixty, but along the way she'd had her share of ailments—a touch of "the sugar" and high blood pressure, along with her breathing problems. In addition to her low energy, she didn't have much of an appetite either.

Sara's daughter Lillian had been asking her mother for some time to go in for more complete tests. "I'm worried about your heart, Mama. You know that heart trouble runs in the family." But Sara felt she was doing reasonably well for a woman her age. And she didn't choose to see any more doctors than she had to.

As Sara got up to make her coffee and put her mind to the Thanksgiving dinner she'd cook that day, the phone rang. She was certain it was Lillian, who knew her hours and didn't hesitate to call early. Lillian was her pride and joy, a lawyer, happily married to a man who owned a small hi-tech business that Sara never quite completely understood. It was enough for her to know they loved one another and were doing well. She didn't exactly think of Lillian as a counterweight to the boys, but she was that, and it made her mother happy.

"Mama, just wanted to let you know I'll be over around nine to help you cook."

"You don't need to do that, honey. I enjoy doing it myself."

"I know you do, Mama, but you have to share a little of that pleasure. It's my day off and I need to get my hands into something."

Sara showered and set to peeling apples for the pie. She always liked to do the pies first, one sweet potato and one apple, everyone praising them and having a piece of each. But relaxed as she felt, her breathing was still heavy, so bad that she felt a little light-headed and had to stop what she was doing for a minute and concentrate on catching her breath. By now Bryan was up, getting ready to go to work.

"You know, Ma," he said, drinking his coffee at one end of the table while she did what she could to resume her task at the other, "I made a decision last night. That little house I was looking at on School Street . . . I'm going to buy it. Take a little pressure off you and get my life moving ahead again."

The good news cheered her, but it didn't help her breathing, and when he was gone she went back to her room to lie down a minute. Next thing she knew Lillian was there, worrying over her.

"Mama, what are you doing in bed with your clothes on? You don't look good, and I don't like the sound of your breathing. How long's that been going on?"

Now it all came out—the three months of breathing trouble, too busy caring for the boys to go to the doctor, the whole thing. Lillian, always the decisive one, had Sara bundled and in the car before she could argue.

Sara was one of the lucky ones. Four days of hospital rest, with medication, and she was ready to go home. But she'd be back again before long, the doctor told her and Lillian, if she didn't change her ways. He prescribed medications, a strict diet, and an exercise rehabilitation plan. Sara treated both recommendations with an "I guess so" indifference, but Lillian got the message. "From now on, Mama, you're going to treat yourself as good as you deserve. And if those brothers of mine can't learn to help you care for yourself, you can bet I will."

Her doctor diagnosed Sara's condition as severe congestive heart failure and high blood pressure. He treated her with medications that would help her heart beat more efficiently and more strongly and that would rid her body of the fluid build-up that results from this condition. He also gave her medication to control her high blood pressure.

"Now it's up to you, Sara," the doctor said. "You keep up with the medication, your diet, and your exercise, and between the two of us, I think we can keep you out of the hospital for a good long while."

WHAT IS CONGESTIVE HEART FAILURE?

When the heart can't pump blood efficiently, we call the condition congestive heart failure. You recall that the heart pumps blood through the major artery called the aorta, from which the blood is carried to all the subsidiary (and smaller) arteries that feed oxygen and nutrients to our organs. When the oxygen and nutrients have been extracted, the blood is returned to the heart through channels called veins. The depleted, unoxygenated blood returns to the right side of the heart, where it is pumped into the lungs and reoxygenated. Then the process starts again.

When the heart doesn't pump efficiently (congestive heart failure), the blood flow to the organs diminishes, which can result in organ failure. Liver, lung, kidney, and eventually the heart itself can fail as a result of this condition.

When the heart can't pump blood efficiently, we call the condition congestive heart failure.

WHAT CAUSES CONGESTIVE HEART FAILURE?

The most common cause of congestive heart failure is hypertension (high blood pressure), which, as you now know, is especially widespread in the African American community. Other causes of CHF include coronary artery disease, viral or bacterial infection, and alcohol abuse. Idiopathic congestive heart failure is also a possibility, meaning that doctors can find no clear reason for the heart failure. Finally, congestive heart failure can result from valvular problems in the heart itself. Specifically, the heart's four valves act as one-way doors, allowing blood to enter into one chamber and then into the next, without going backward. When these valves don't open efficiently and that condition goes untreated, congestive heart failure results.

The most common cause of congestive heart failure is hypertension.

WHAT ARE THE SYMPTOMS OF CONGESTIVE HEART FAILURE?

Though congestive heart failure can have any number of different causes, the symptoms are essentially the same.

- Patients have trouble breathing, especially when they exert themselves.
- Patients feel constantly tired and, increasingly, will avoid exercise.
- In the early stages, patients gain weight and look puffy in the face and lower legs.
- Patients often need to sleep upright or with the support of a pillow to improve their breathing. (This is because blood backs up into the lungs and makes breathing difficult.)
- Patients in advanced stages of this condition lack appetite and organ function and lose a lot of weight. This symptom, called "cardiac wasting," is caused by the slow dying off of the organs.

CONGESTIVE HEART FAILURE AND THE AFRICAN AMERICAN COMMUNITY

The facts are shocking: African American men are two times as likely to die of CHF than white men. African American women are two and a half to three times more likely to die of CHF than white women. Although poorer medical treatment as the result of socioeconomic differences is to blame for some of this increased rate of CHF among African Americans, even once such factors have been taken into account, African Americans are still much more susceptible, and more likely, to die of CHF than whites. Consider these facts:

- The high rate of hypertension in the African American community is the number one reason for CHF among this population. Uncontrolled hypertension can lead not only to coronary artery disease but to congestive heart failure.
- Uncontrolled diabetes—another widespread condition in the African American community—is the second main cause for CHF.
- Alcohol abuse contributes to CHF because alcohol in excessive quantities poisons and permanently damages the heart cells.
- Obesity, especially among African American women, can contribute to CHF.
- Cigarette smoking can lead to CHF.
- Chronic stress is a major problem. As we explain later in more detail, your nervous system is hyperactive in times of stress. Part of that hyperactivity results in a faster and more intense heartbeat, as you've probably experienced yourself in moments of extreme emotion. Such hyperactivity can be dangerous to a heart that is already failing.

African American men are two times as likely to die of CHF than white men. African women are 2 1/2–3 times more likely to die of CHF than white women.

African Americans are more likely than whites to be victims of CHF because they are less likely to be diagnosed and treated for it. The reasons for this situation are complex. Where there is poverty there is obviously less access to medical care. Sometimes the problem is a lack of knowledge about this disease and therefore failure to recognize it as a disease.

Women like Sara may remain untreated simply because they consider their own well-being and health care less important than the health of their loved ones. Such a stance may be considered noble or necessary to the family's survival. We've all known young and old African American mothers who ignored their own health needs because their babies needed shoes or important bills had to be paid. Obviously, there's no easy solution to conflicts like these: When there isn't enough time or money to go around, people make choices, and many good people give of themselves freely, sometimes without taking adequate care of themselves.

To assume that African Americans are somehow less worthy of medical treatment than whites is to submit to a kind of prejudice—indeed, it is to impose that prejudice and disrespect on ourselves.

But to ignore your health because you can't afford the time or the money necessary to attend to it seems to us short-sighted. Too often it leads to eventual incapacitation. Sometimes, thinking about yourself is the best way to serve others, and even the poor, armed with knowledge, can get necessary treatment through emergency rooms or free clinics.

The last reason for high mortality rates caused by CHF is one we have returned to often in this book. Many African Americans take a stoic attitude toward our health. Older people may feel that a weakening heart is the inevitable price of old age, or that strong as they are, they can do all right even with a failing heart. Sometimes that strength or stoicism has served our community well, giving us the courage to endure in the face of incredible adversity. But in medical matters it has cost us dearly. Ignoring your health or not taking advantage of medical treatments that are available can be a form of slow suicide. To assume that African Americans are somehow less worthy of medical treatment than whites is to submit to a kind of prejudice—indeed, it is to impose prejudice and disrespect on ourselves. We'd like to think that this book might lead to a kind of "improve yourself through knowledge" movement in the health care of the African American community.

TREATMENT OF CONGESTIVE HEART FAILURE

The starting point for treating CHF is to control the risk factors—that is, hypertension, alcohol consumption, diabetes, obesity, and cigarette smoking. There are also specific medical and nonmedical treatments to alleviate the condition itself. The aim of all the treatments is to strengthen the heart. Once that's done, the symptoms usually take care of themselves.

Changes in Lifestyle

As is so often the case, the heart of the matter is lifestyle and attitudes. Here are some changes you can make today to strengthen your heart and lessen the likelihood of contracting CHF:

- Decrease sodium intake to 2 to 3 grams a day. That means not simply cutting down on added salt but also checking the salt content of processed foods.

- Exercise. The heart is a muscle that needs to be worked. Exercise will strengthen the heart and make it more durable. (*Caution:* If you already suffer from CHF or show any of the symptoms, consult your doctor before beginning an exercise program. He or she can tell you what level of exercise is appropriate.)
- Avoid excessive fluid intake. If you suffer from CHF, the heart is inclined toward fluid overload, "water on the lungs," or pulmonary edema, and that condition leads to labored breathing.
- Control alcohol consumption.
- Don't smoke.
- Take medications for high blood pressure and diabetes if they have been prescribed, and don't stop taking them unless so ordered by your doctor.
- Control your weight.
- Visit your doctor regularly.

Nonsurgical Medical Treatment

Several drugs and classes of drugs can effectively treat CHF. Diuretics, or water pills, force our bodies to urinate excess water that otherwise causes congestion, fluid overload, and weight gain. By controlling the buildup of excess fluid, diuretics help strengthen the heart. If you are taking diuretics, it is essential that you have your potassium level monitored, because diuretics deplete the body not only of water but of potassium and sodium as well. Your doctor will prescribe potassium supplements to maintain the proper balance.

By controlling the buildup of excess fluid, diuretics strengthen the heart.

Another group of drugs commonly prescribed to treat CHF are the vasodilators. These drugs dilate, or widen, the arteries that carry blood to the heart, thus helping the heart to work better. Remember that the heart pumps blood through the aorta into the smaller arteries. The wider these arteries are, the easier blood flows through them and the less the heart has to work.

Another group of drugs used effectively are ACE (angiotensin converting enzyme) inhibitors. Like vasodilators, these inhibitors also dilate the arteries coming from the aorta. Though it isn't clear why, ACE inhibitors have been proven especially effective in treating CHF in African American patients.

ACE inhibitors have proven especially effective in treating CHF in African American patients.

Here, too, certain cautions need to be observed. ACE inhibitors can cause kidney failure, so your doctor should monitor your kidney function. These inhibitors can also cause fluctuations in your blood pressure, so that too needs to be carefully monitored. Finally, some patients suffer persistent coughing when using ACE inhibitors. If that symptom becomes severe, your doctor will either change the dosage or put you on another drug.

Digoxin or Lanoxin has proven effective in some cases, by strengthening the heart's ability to squeeze, and therefore to pump, more effectively.

Finally, the beta blockers have proven useful in treating CHF. Beta blockers, as their name suggests, block beta receptors on the heart. Such receptors are similar to mailboxes: When the mail carrier delivers a letter, we read it and the message determines how we respond. The heart's receptors, called beta receptors, receive chemical messages that tell the heart to speed up or slow down. Beta blockers specifically block those receptors that cause the heart to speed up, thus allowing the heart to conserve energy and work more effectively.

Beta blockers will not ordinarily be prescribed to patients in acute stages of CHF or to patients with severe lung problems such as emphysema or asthma. A beta blocker slows the heart and makes it beat less vigorously—obviously not the effect we want when the patient has severe or critical CHF and his or her heart is already working very poorly.

Surgical Treatment

Bypass surgery, angioplasty (ballooning of the artery), or stent placement can relieve CHF if it's caused by underlying coronary artery disease. (Angioplasty and stent replacement are included here to distinguish them from medical treatments. Technically, they are non-surgical.) All these treatments improve CHF by increasing the flow of blood to the heart. See chapter 3 for explanations of these procedures.

Surgical treatment can also help if the CHF is caused by problems with the valves of the heart. When the valves do not open effectively, the heart will begin to fail and ultimately CHF will result. In such cases, surgery is usually the best and most long-lasting treatment. Even for patients at critical stages of CHF, surgery can offer relief.

Cardiac transplantation is a treatment of last resort used only when bypass surgery, angioplasty, or stenting doesn't work. Its success depends on the patient's general medical condition, and organs available for transplant are always in short supply.

A heart transplant may give a patient a second chance at life. Patient's have an 85-90% chance of surviving the first five years after a transplant. But that survival period is sometimes difficult. The drugs necessary to prevent the body from rejecting the transplanted heart can have dangerous side effects—including increased risk of infection, kidney failure, and pulmonary problems.

Another surgical treatment for CHF is called left ventricular assist device (or LVAD). This device, a miniature pump connected to the heart and aorta by surgery, helps the heart work better by doing much of the heart's work. Not a long term remedy in itself, the LVAD is rather a bridge for those awaiting transplantation.

Finally, a new form of laser surgery, referred to as TMR, or transmyocardial revascularization, has been found effective in some cases. In this procedure, minute holes are made with a laser in the heart itself to increase the blood flow to the heart muscle. This still somewhat experimental procedure is performed only at hospitals designated as heart centers.

Chapter 8

HYPERTENSION: AN AFRICAN AMERICAN EPIDEMIC

ALTHOUGH IT WAS NEARLY seven years since her husband had died, every day something brought it back. On this morning, a Sunday in May, it was Luther Vandross singing "Here and Now" on the clock-radio. Waking, Amy Cross remembered Andrew singing it to her on their wedding day. For a moment, listening to the song, she slipped out of the present and tasted the sweetness of the past. Then, as it always did, the sweetness dissolved into the terrible memory of the day she took the call from an emergency room doctor telling her that her husband of five years was dead.

Andrew's death was a bolt from the blue. Despite her parents' warnings, Amy had married this forty-year-old man when she was only twenty-two. Before she married him, she knew that he had high blood pressure, but neither she nor Andrew thought much about it. With Amy's help, Andrew took his blood pressure medication regularly and stuck to a low-fat, low-cholesterol, and low-salt diet. He did what the doctor told him. Shouldn't that have been enough?

Hypertension—high blood pressure—is a major killer in the African American community, and a major cause of hypertension is stress. Amy knew that all too well and couldn't help but feel anger—and, with it, her own blood pressure was rising. Wasn't Andrew just another victim of institutionalized racism? Wasn't his constant expectation of racial snubs, his paranoia as they both called it, itself a symptom of the real snubs and insults that he ran into every day? "That's just the thing, baby," he'd said to her more than once. "How can you, how can any of us, separate the real from the imagined, when we get slapped repeatedly with the real?"

Hypertension is a major killer in the African American community.

He'd often bring the dilemma to the dinner table. "He only looked at me that way because I was black. . . . He wouldn't have said that to me if I was white. . . . I'd have gotten that promotion if I was white."

Andrew was an ambitious man. But he was also, Amy was convinced, an amiable one. When she saw him, relaxed, playing with the baby, joking with their friends, walking on the beach with her, hand in hand, she knew she was seeing the man God had intended him to be. But Andrew could never learn to take in stride the daily pressure of being black in America. Amy had tried to teach him how to do that. "Racism is like gravity," she'd tell him. "You just have to live with it." Instead, he'd died of its effects, and now, as she lay there thinking for the thousandth time about his death, she wondered if she and their son might not die of it too.

This was the day Amy would graduate from law school, the day she began to imagine for herself a year after Andrew's death. With a child to raise, not much money, and a less than brilliant college career behind her, she had enrolled in a community college to take courses she needed to get her on track. Within a year she'd won admission to law school, though sometimes she felt half drowned by the pressures she was under. Now, on this Sunday, she was reaping the harvest.

But the harvest included some bitterness. The stories that Andrew had told her about the workplace had begun to ring true for her also. Sitting alone, the only African American woman in the class, she often felt invisible to the professors, to the other students. Or, after class, when she cornered a professor to ask a question about some case she'd read or he'd referred to, she'd been made to feel that he was too busy to talk to her, that she was wasting his time. Because she was black? Because he was arrogant and didn't take seriously his job as a teacher? In any case, the result was the same. She felt frustrated, dejected, and unsure of herself. Only the stubborn will and strength she shared with so many African American women had allowed her to go on. She refused to quit.

Often, studying late at night, after hours of classes and work at the check-out counter of the grocery store, after she'd put young AJ to bed, she thought that if she had the privilege of being a full-time student, she'd be number one in her class. She was still among the top dozen, and she felt certain that she'd be a damn good lawyer. But she knew that it wouldn't matter how good she was if she couldn't handle stress—Andrew's death had taught her this.

On graduation morning, as she dressed in front of the mirror and noted the extra weight she'd put on during these stressful years when she had no time to take care of herself, she made a resolution. She'd get back in shape and stay there. She'd raise their son not only to a life of opportunity but to a life of health and emotional balance. Today was a red-letter day. She'd graduate from law school. But she was graduating, that very morning, into a new way of thinking. She would not let stress kill her or her son as it had killed the man she loved.

Consider the following facts about stress:

- People suffering from chronic stress are 4.5 times more likely to die of heart attack or stroke.
- Many adult visits to doctors are for stress-related illnesses.
- Job stress in the United States, with its attendant absenteeism, lost productivity, and insurance claims, costs approximately $200 billion annually.
- In a 1995 poll, seven of ten people interviewed said that they felt stress in a typical workday, and 43 percent reported that they suffered physical and emotional symptoms of burnout.

THE HARMFUL EFFECTS OF STRESS

Let's talk about what stress is and what it does to the body. From an evolutionary point of view, stress is a protective mechanism. It allows the body to rise to its utmost performance in response to some immediate danger. So it is when an otherwise tranquil female black bear turns savage in response to a real or imagined threat to her cubs. So it is when a fish in a stream suddenly swims away, frightened by your shadow. And so it is with you when, in an emergency, you experience absolute clarity and become capable of extraordinary action, as your body seems to say, "Let me handle this. We don't have time to think about it."

Though the immediate stress reaction is a kind of ultimate performance enhancer, it's also very strong medicine that is meant to be taken only in real emergencies. Unfortunately, for the chronically stressed person, this emergency response system is operating much of the time, even all of the time. And when that happens, stress can bring nothing but harm.

When the brain interprets the outside environment as dangerous, it signals for the production by the adrenal gland of hormones called *cortisol* and *epinephrine* (epinephrine is commonly known as adrenaline). Cortisol helps regulate metabolism and immunity, while epinephrine helps activate our central nervous system, at the same time increasing the heart rate and quickening the breathing. But while these are some of the specific responses, when cortisol and epinepherine are flowing during times of stress, they affect every part of your body.

In situations of real danger, this chemical response can save your life. When your brain interprets a stimulus as dangerous, a number of events take place quickly. For one, the body suppresses pain. At the same time, brain functions—memory, thinking itself—are improved: Your thinking is sharper and clearer and more precise. Other changes take place as well. Your heart beats faster, your blood pressure rises, your muscles tense, and your senses sharpen. Your eyes dilate for better vision and your lungs take in more oxygen, preparing your body for action. Your liver is busy producing extra glucose, which creates more energy, so your heart beats faster and more powerfully, improving the blood flow. Your spleen also is in overdrive, producing more blood cells than usual in order to transport the extra oxygen taken in by the lungs. Even the hairs on your body become erect in response to the flow of epinephrine.

In situations of physical danger, such stress reactions save lives. Even when you are faced with some unusually demanding task, stress can sometimes help you rise to efforts you didn't think you had in you. Healthy people are familiar with the way they can transform stress, and even fear, into exceptional performance. But problems result when this emergency reactive system becomes chronic. Then your body's inability to perform continually at this high level of intensity may result in unwelcome symptoms, either physical or emotional—and often both. The physical symptoms can include:

- Overeating
- Disturbed motor skills
- Weight gain or excessive weight loss
- Diarrhea or constipation
- Sleeplessness
- Headaches
- Hyperactivity

- Hyperventilation
- Sexual problems
- Excessive drinking
- Drug or nicotine dependence

Emotional symptoms can include:

- Anxiety
- Anger
- Agitation
- Insecurity
- Depression or feelings of worthlessness
- Paranoia
- Denial, in the form of refusing to take responsibility for your behavior
- Suicidal tendencies
- Lack of satisfaction from happy activities
- Avoiding work and putting things off
- Excessive gambling
- Overexaggeration or overcompensation, in the form of arrogance, swagger, hostility, or other kinds of acting out
- Spending excessively on inessential material things
- Irresponsibility

Mental symptoms can include:

- Forgetfulness
- Reduced creativity

- Inability to concentrate
- Preoccupation with the past rather than the present and future

Unfortunately we all have acquaintances, even family members, who have become victims to alcoholism, drugs, excessive gambling or shopping, compulsive sexual promiscuity, or other addictive behaviors. We know promising and productive people who mysteriously slip, crash, and end up as drug addicts, alcoholics, or prostitutes. Often, when you look at such cases closely enough, the reasons for the crash become less mysterious: Falling off the right path is frequently the result of stress that you're incapable of coping with. The result may be emotional and physical ruin.

No matter where you live or how, there's stress enough to go around. Stress is absolutely democratic.

Stress-related suffering isn't confined to situations of obvious stress. You don't have to be CEO of a Fortune 500 company, or an airline traffic controller, or a cardiac surgeon, to experience it. A bright young woman caught in a dead-end job, a single working mother trying to get educated (a person like Amy), a father rushing home from work to pick up his daughter at day care—we have all felt it. No matter where you live or how, there's enough stress to go around. Stress is absolutely democratic. It comes with our desire to perform well, to be better, and to achieve; it comes with marriage and child raising; it's in our family relations, in our day-to-day efforts to be nice to others.

But while some measure of stress is universal, African Americans usually experience extra large portions. Because racism and discrimination are institutionalized, it's often difficult to know if the hard time that your boss is giving you is directed against your performance or your skin color. When you walk into a well-lit bank at noon to make a deposit for the company you own and the woman standing in front of you clutches her purse close to her, is it because she's nervous and would do this when anyone came up behind her, or because you are black? You know that in these cases what makes for chronic stress isn't the certainty that you are being met with bigotry. It's the uncertainty.

Chronic stress, as we've seen, is harmful to the body and the soul. It can even weaken the immune system. Researchers at Carnegie Mellon University found that people experiencing high stress were twice as likely to get colds. (The assumption is that the hormones triggered by stress inhibit the function of the white cells to fight off disease.) The adrenal glands themselves suffer from prolonged stress, and the heavy secretions of cortisol (which, with adrenaline, are produced by the adrenal glands) can become toxic when they are produced steadily. Chronic stress can lead to the body's inability to break down (that is, metabolize) glucose, a failure that leads to diabetes. And the decreased blood flow to the intestines can lead to ulcers. Finally, coming home to the subject of this book, chronic stress is linked closely with hypertension, along with the coronary disease and congestive heart failure that often follow from it.

Chronic stress can make you susceptible to diseases ranging from the common cold to diabetes and ulcers. It is also linked closely with heart disease.

Chronic stress also affects the way we think—and don't think. Fatigue, anger, and depression weaken our mental functions. Thus, a common stereotype of the angry or uptight African American that we see often—far too often—on television has a grain of truth in it. It's not because we are born that way but because chronic stress can often lead to such states.

By elevating the blood pressure and causing hypertension, stress leads to coronary artery disease. It also causes the heart rate to increase, and that overwork in itself can lead to heart failure.

Finally, chronic stress has a variety of bad effects on the coronary system and the heart itself. By elevating the blood pressure and causing hypertension, stress leads to coronary artery disease. It also causes the heart rate to increase, and that overwork in itself can lead to heart failure. Because stress damages the elasticity of blood vessels, it can lead to the development of plaque, which, as you now know, can obstruct a coronary artery and cause coronary artery disease. The chemicals released by stress may increase the tendency toward elevated cholesterol and fat in the bloodstream, a condition that may result in coronary artery disease and even heart attacks. And, as you also know, stress can lead to obesity, another major risk factor in the development of coronary artery disease, just as it may encourage smoking and alcoholism, also major risk factors. In combination, these problems are especially deadly.

DEPRESSION

A major ailment that results from stress is depression. We'll call it a psychosomatic ailment, because it's a disease of the mind that also deeply involves the body. In the African American community depression tends to be overlooked and under-reported—in part because it's often seen as a sign of weakness or as a sign that the victim has lost faith in God or in life itself. These reasons, sometimes combined with the terrible impact of poverty and lack of knowledge that can accompany it, mean that in the African American community stress and depression too often go untreated. That's especially unfortunate, because there are now a number of ways, ranging from counseling to medication, to treat depression effectively.

In the African American community stress and depression too often go untreated.

Most of us are familiar with the signs and symptoms of depression, but if you're one of the fortunate ones who isn't, here they are:

- Irritability and chronic fatigue
- Sleeping too much or too little
- Heavy reliance on alcohol and drugs, including nicotine
- Inability to concentrate or make decisions
- Feelings of worthlessness and guilt, sometimes played out as hostility and anger
- Inability to act, even when action is necessary

Depression often follows stress that we can't cope with. The inability to cope in turn causes feelings of worthlessness. And so the terrible spiral plunges. The depressed person, besides falling into addictions to drugs, stimulants, or even food, will experience abnormally high levels of adrenal secretions, which can lead to high blood pressure and, eventually, coronary disease.

In the next chapter we talk at length about ways to control stress and the accompanying depression. For the time being, let's simply say that help is available—first, from counseling, whether by a psychologist or by a minister, pastor, or priest; second, through new medications; and, finally, through a variety of self-help programs of exercise and meditation that millions of people have discovered can change their lives. Sadly, African Americans are underexposed to these new and effective therapies.

SOCIAL ISOLATION

If depression goes untreated, the social isolation African Americans often experience outside their community can become progressively worse. Social isolation may be forced on us in the classroom, in the streets, in shops, or in the boardroom. It's a vicious circle.

Many studies have established that the absence of a social support system is in itself a risk factor that contributes to coronary artery disease, hypertension, and stroke. This has been especially documented among women who isolate themselves, whether as a result of general depression, or because of the direct loss of a spouse or loved one. These studies find that married people suffer fewer heart attacks than single or widowed people. And older people, long married, who suffer the loss of a spouse, though they themselves are in apparently good health, often die soon afterward. So it's not just in fairy tales that people die of broken hearts. In real life, too, grief and loss—and isolation—can result in heart disease and a higher death rate.

Naturally, the most effective cure for isolation is to get involved with family and friends—to reestablish connections with a social group. Admittedly, for older persons, or for younger ones suffering depression, such moves aren't always easy. Sometimes we can build up to the needed interaction. Isolated people who have pets live longer than those who don't. And they have less heart disease. Here, what common sense tells us is the best guide. We weren't made to be alone. Whatever it takes, we must do what we can to connect—with people, if possible, or, in a pinch, with dogs, cats, even with fish in an aquarium.

Another form of social isolation that's often harmful to the heart is conceit, or excessive self-involvement, as surprising as that may be. Studies of heart patients at the University of California at San Francisco[2] found that they were especially likely to use pronouns such as I, me, and mine. Excessive self-involvement is a risk factor for coronary artery disease, because it can cause high blood pressure. Egotistic people are more likely than others to quickly show hostility and anger, and those behaviors work to isolate these people further.

Well, maybe it shouldn't be a surprise. The good, the generous, and the happy live longer than the hostile and self-absorbed. It's not always easy to be good, to care for others more than we care for ourselves, to stay connected. And Lord knows that it isn't always easy to be happy. But the odd fact is that, along with the spiritual benefits, those who can cast bread upon the waters are likely to live longer than those who don't.

---

2 See Linda Ojeda, Ph.D., *Her Healthy Heart: A Woman's Guide to Preventing and Reversing Heart Disease Naturally* [Hunter House, 1998], pp. 62-63)

Chapter 9

STRESS RELIEF FOR AFRICAN AMERICANS

AS HE DRESSED, Ronald Lloyd Lewis was still riding the wave of happiness that broke over him when Dr. Gant, his cardiologist, said he could go home. Ronald had been in the hospital for five days to recover from a moderately severe heart attack, and all that time he'd feared he would have to undergo surgery. But now that Dr. Gant had studied Ronald's complete cardiac workup, he'd concluded that Ronald didn't require bypass surgery, angioplasty, or stenting. "For what ails you, Ronald, medication will do the job. Medication, a better diet, and some work at stress reduction, because that's what it's going to take to keep you out of my hands."

Even that warning hadn't clouded Ronald's spirits. It was a beautiful day, he was alive, his wife would be with him any moment, and he was going home. And he'd already concluded, even before Dr. Gant made his report, that he had to change his life. He'd never loved life so much as he did at this moment.

Ronald had a lot to love. A highly successful lawyer, he'd also enjoyed political success. He'd already served a term in the state legislature and now friends were urging him to run for Congress. His two daughters gave him great joy. Tonya was already in college, preparing to follow in his footsteps, and Jasmine would enroll in two years.

But there were shadows in his life, as there are in everyone's. He worried a little about what his wife Adrienne would do once Jasmine went off to school. He worried about whether to enter the congressional race, with the enormous demands it would make on his time and his money, and the necessity, if he won, of spending less time with his family because he would be in Washington much of the time. And, of course, with one daughter in college and another close to entering, money was always on his mind. But running deeper than the worry was the wild confidence he'd always enjoyed. He was born to lead the pack.

Ronald remembered how, after two hours of sleep, he had driven back from a late-night meeting and had been seized by a rush of adrenaline. Racing at speeds up to ninety-five miles per hour, he'd passed everyone on the road, and when he finally pulled into the garage at three A.M. he had that old feeling of victory. He'd won another race and he actually imagined the victory flag waving.

Remembering that moment, Ronald had a new thought. Had he been running after something all his life or was he being chased? In the aftermath of his brush with death, he saw the answer clearly. Always, beneath his energy and confidence, his willingness to handle not only his own problems but the problems of everyone around him, there was a naked fear of inadequacy. At this stage of his life it was too late to say whether that fear was something born in him with his skin color or if it came from somewhere else altogether. Certainly, being a black man in America, riding the history of slavery and humiliation, skin color had a lot to do with it. But he also understood enough about human beings to see that, under all the masks that people wear to hide it, this fear of inadequacy was universal. The real question wasn't how to get rid of it but how to tame it and use it to his advantage.

Fear of inadequacy is universal. The real question isn't how to get rid of it but how to tame it and use it to your advantage.

Ronald was a strong believer in God, and phrases he'd heard repeatedly in church rang in his head now: "Ever have any doubt? The Lord will surely bring you out! . . . He will never let you down. . . ." And he'd always drawn great comfort from this passage in Proverbs: "Trust in the Lord with all thine heart; and lean not unto thine own understanding. In all thy ways acknowledge Him and He shall direct thy paths." But today the phrases weren't enough. And for a moment the joy he'd felt at the prospect of returning home darkened into fear. He'd lived through this heart attack, but what if there were a second? He saw someone else assuming his partnership in the firm. He saw another man holding his wife. He imagined his children growing into adult life without him at their side. And he knew that he had a new race to run, harder than all the others. Now he must learn to slow down and to make that inner peace that had always eluded him.

Even at his moments of purest triumph, he now saw that a lurking sense of inadequacy never left him. Instead, it made demands. No sooner had he finished a job, climbed a mountain, than it whispered, "Well that couldn't have been much of a challenge, could it, since a worthless guy like you met it? When are you going to accomplish something really big—something *real*?"

Then Ronald knew he had an answer to this. He was going to learn the tricks of managing that endlessly accusing, endlessly negative voice. The Lord hadn't put him into the world just to be a high hurdler. He was 54 years old—old enough to grow up. And somehow, he sensed, that meant giving up an illusion that he'd held dear all his life—the illusion that he controlled his life and his destiny—an illusion he'd managed to hold onto despite his true and deep faith in God.

STRESS MANAGEMENT

Thanks to numerous studies, we know a lot about stress today. We know that stress is a social evil that carries with it great expense in terms of the cost of illness and loss of productivity. We know that, on a more human scale, stress means physical suffering for many of us. And it means, too, for many more, that life loses its savor, because our experience comes to us through the screen of anxiety.

The first step in managing stress is to know when and why we are stressed.

Happily, we also know a good deal about stress management. We speak of "management" rather than "cure" because it doesn't look as if stress can be cured. It comes with the territory for all of us—black or white, rich or poor. So the question is, how do we best learn to live with it? Here are some tips.

We must examine when and why we are stressed. Sometimes that's easy. You're in a hurry to get somewhere and the car in front of you remains at the stoplight after it has turned green. The driver is so wrapped up in his cell phone conversation that he's forgotten he's in a car. This is a moment when you're prepared to make yourself feel bad, by letting your anger take over. Why is this guy doing this to you? The driver becomes, at that moment, an embodiment of everything that's wrong with the world, everything that works against you. Even if you don't voice that anger, it's easy to let the feeling take over and to abruptly find yourself in the nasty world that rage shapes for all of us. That world is nasty not only psychologically but physically as well, because it is made of stress. The more often we slip into it, the more harm we do to ourselves.

For most of us, these situations may be relatively easy to cope with. We accept them as inescapable irritations in the business of moving through life each day with other human beings. In one way or another, somebody is likely to bump into us—on purpose or inadvertently. There is, however, another way you can accept the bumps and bruises—with a kind of humor. Indeed, laughter is the best medicine for stress. It works very well against the tendency we all have to think catastrophically—that is, to make small problems bigger by latching onto them.

Keep a stress diary

There are other effective ways to keep stress from controlling our lives. You might want to keep a stress diary for a couple of weeks, recording the things that set you off, and describing your own reactions to them. It's a way of getting a little perspective on the cause of the stress. At the same time, cultivate physical disciplines that help you defend against stress. When you sense yourself about to "go off," practice deep and steady breathing. If you feel yourself going tense, deliberately relax the muscles that are tense. You'll be surprised how your mood can change. And here's another tip: Try smiling. It's an odd trick the body has. If we put on a countenance of happiness, the actual happiness tends to follow. Try it. It works.

The worst way to suffer stress is in isolation. Because stress can mean self-obsession, depression, and feelings of worthlessness, people suffering stress may often find themselves pulling away from family and friends. Or their hostile behaviors may drive others away. We're social animals, after all, and there are a number of ways to renew our sense of positive human relationship.

Go to a park where there are children. Watching them play, hearing them laugh, can be terrific medicine. Call friends to have a meal together. We all know how easy it is to slip into unhappiness when the phone doesn't ring. Well, sometimes you can snap out of your sense of isolation simply by initiating contact with others. An evening with friends can remind us of how much the give and take with others can bring us out of our brooding and into the sun, freeing us from the stress that flourishes when we isolate ourselves.

Sometimes, too, when the situation that stresses you is overwhelming, talking with others can be a way of seeing it more clearly and putting it in perspective. Remember that in many stressful situations it's not advice that we need. Simply by giving words to our suffering or worry, we may begin to see a way out of it.

Stress on the job, as we've seen, is a big problem. And we don't pretend you can always do much about it. A dead-end repetitive job under a bullying (or, sometimes, sexist or racist) boss can be a true nightmare, and sometimes there's nothing else to do but to learn new skills or sharpen the ones you have and look for a new job.

But insofar as the job allows, you often can improve things for yourself. For most people, what causes stress on the job is the feeling of powerlessness. Where possible, then, be an active citizen in the workplace. Ask questions and make suggestions. And cultivate good relationships with fellow workers. Sometimes that sense of solidarity can be the beginning of a renewed sense of control.

Experts urge you to be decisive and assertive at work. How do I get there from here? you may ask. Simply writing down what the problem is and a list of your options for solving it—even the option of doing nothing—can be an excellent start. List not only the obvious solutions but also the unusual ones; and for each, list their pros and cons. Sometimes, through such a process, you discover that problems that seemed to have no solutions actually have several. Play with those solutions. Be flexible, keeping in mind that if you decide on one and it doesn't pay off, you can turn to another. The mere activity of working toward a solution will bring its own rewards. Action, in such matters, is nearly always preferable to inaction, and clear and patient thought can be a form of action.

Experts urge you to make yourself decisive and assertive.

By the same token, get into the habit of saying what you think, knowing what you want, and doing what's in your power to get it. This doesn't mean you have to become a loudmouth or a bully. It means you must have self-respect. In the process of expressing your views, you'll find that others will express theirs to you. You may find yourself changing, or others changing under your influence. Start conversations. Initiate friendships. You may be out of practice and feel rusty. But, as in all things, practice will make, if not perfect, better. It's just a question of persistence.

Get into the habit of saying what you think, knowing what you want, and getting what's in your power to get.

And knowing what you want is the first step toward getting it. Sometimes we sink so deeply into stress-related depression that we feel too powerless to want anything. Though in that state any motion is difficult, try making a list of ten things you like to do. Make other lists of things you'd like to see happen in your life. Stay focused and keep your eyes on the big picture—even when, as Dr. Martin Luther King Jr. put it, "the cup of endurance runs over."

STRESS, DIET, AND VITAMINS

We've talked about diet in another context. But in matters of stress, too, it matters enormously what you eat. In 1997, the *New England Journal of Medicine*[1] published a study called "Dietary Approaches to Stop Hypertension," known as DASH. The study found that a low-fat diet high in calcium, along with plenty of fruits and vegetables, significantly helped lower blood pressure in people of all races. But, remarkably, the benefit of such a diet was twice as great in African Americans. In fact, the DASH diet low-

1 Appel, L. J. et al., "A Clinical Trial of the Effects of Dietary Patterns on Blood Pressure," *New England Journal of Medicine*, 336[16], April 17, 1997; 1117-24.

ered the blood pressure of the test just as effectively as did blood pressure medications. So ask your doctor about the DASH diet. Or check it out yourself by consulting the website: www.dash/.bwh.harvard.edu; or by calling 800-575-WELL. You might find that this diet improves both your health and your outlook on life.

Whatever diet you choose, it's essential that you avoid junk food when you are stressed. You'd be wise also to avoid alcohol, nicotine, caffeine, and sugar. Though it is tempting to turn to such stimulants for temporary relief, in fact they aggravate stress. Your doctor may also suggest that you avoid white flour and dairy products, while you increase your intake of raw fruits and vegetables.

What needs most to be emphasized here is that to control hypertension by changing the way we eat means a lifelong commitment. It does not require that you totally eliminate fat—simply, that you eat a balanced and healthy diet.

Because stress depletes the vitamins in the body and that depletion can worsen depression, anxiety, insomnia, and stomach upsets, you will need to concentrate not simply on diet but also on getting enough of the right vitamins. Your doctor may recommend vitamin supplements.

Stress depletes the vitamins in the body.

The B complex vitamins are especially helpful for repairing damage to the immune system, reducing anxiety, and improving brain function. Your doctor may recommend an intramuscular injection, which provides quick relief for some people. Or he may suggest that you take B complex vitamins in tablet form.

Vitamins A and C, and E are effective antioxidants. Free radicals are generated during stress, and the antioxidants are useful in destroying these.

Your doctor may also suggest supplemental doses of calcium, magnesium, and potassium, each of which can help repair damage brought on by stress.

While recommended dosages can be found in books like Dr. James F. Balch's *Prescriptions for Nutritional Healing*[2], consult with your doctor before you begin a vitamin supplement plan. He can instruct you about the possibilities and dangers of overdose, and ensure that your vitamin schedule is consistent with your medical condition. Pregnant women must be especially cautious about high vitamin intake.

SLEEP

Certainly if you're sleepless because of stress, you need to correct the problem. Sleeplessness feeds stress and makes you moody, angry, more vulnerable to illness and to the things that caused you stress in the first place. Regulating your sleep should be a top priority.

Make regulating your sleep a top priority.

That means avoiding stimulants like alcohol, caffeine, and nicotine. All of them can disrupt sleep. Develop good habits for getting ready to sleep. If you watch a violent movie before going to bed, you're not likely to slip easily into sleep. Find ways to calm your-

2 James F. Balch, *Prescriptions for Nutritional Healing.* Avery Publishing Group: 2nd ed., 1998.

self before bed. Read something that soothes or even bores you. Listen to mellow music. Once in bed, remove the obvious obstacles to sleep. Use ear plugs to eliminate annoying noise. Relax your body by methodically tensing and then relaxing muscles—first your feet, then gradually up your legs, the trunk of your body, your chest, neck, jaw, cheeks, and brow. Do it a few times if necessary. It works.

Giving attention to your breathing can also help. Try to steady and slow it. Give your attention to your breath. When your mind wanders, bring it back, gently, to the breath.

If none of this helps, other resources are available. Ask your doctor to refer you to a sleep clinic where you can get medical treatment or treatment through biofeedback. We do *not* recommend over-the-counter sleep enhancers. If you are suffering sleep problems, self-medication can be risky. Best talk to your doctor.

PRAYER AND MEDITATION

Turning the mind to something or someone larger than the self is a proven and effective way of coping with stress. (Interestingly, the biblical Psalms are the highest model we have of prayer as stress relief. Philippians 4:6-7 and Isaiah 26:3 both offer direct comfort to those in stress.) The cardiologist Dr. Randolph Byrd reports[3] that patients who pray daily are less likely to be sick than those who do not pray, and, if they become sick, the sickness will be less severe. Others have found that prayer can reduce high

---

3 Randolph C. Byrd, "Positive Therapeutic Effects of Intercessory Prayer in a Coronary Care Unit Population," *Southern Medical Journal* 81:7 (1988).

Patients who pray daily are less likely to be sick, and, if sick, to suffer the sickness less severely, than those who do not.

blood pressure and headaches, ease anxiety and stress, and even help in wound healing.

And while prayer offers those practical benefits, it offers other advantages as well. To keep in contact with a higher power is to acknowledge that we do not carry the weight of the world alone but can share that burden. It tips us toward faith and toward the conviction that our destiny is a positive one. What we recommend here is not doctrinal. For those who are ready to believe, prayer will work its healing, whether the path is Christian, Jewish, Muslim, or Buddhist. Pray for strength, for peace, for healing. Pray not only for yourself but for those you love. And if anger and stress—distress—seem to be driving your life, tell God about this. It can be a first step toward gaining the necessary perspective on destructive forces that threaten you.

As part of a larger network of belief and practice, prayer can bring us into community and into service. Social isolation is the great nourisher of stress, and prayer can lead to greater generosity of self and involvement with others. Attending a church, getting involved in Sunday school or in other forms of service or social activity, are in themselves ways of connecting with something bigger and more important than yourself.

Another important spiritual discipline for managing stress is meditation. Millions of Americans have found in it a practical exercise that calms them and allows them to taste life's fruits more fully. These days, in major cities, meditation centers are easy to find, and many of them offer free or inexpensive instruction. But the basic principles of meditation are simple enough, and you can begin them without instruction.

Pick a time of day and a place reasonably quiet and free from distractions and interruptions. Sit on a thick cushion on the floor, legs crossed, or in a straight-backed chair, keeping an upright posture so that your back is not supported by the back of the chair. Your spine, your neck, and the top of your head should all be in a line, as though someone were pulling you up with a string attached to the top of your head. In other words, sit tall.

Sit still, resting your hands palms down on your thighs. Rest your eyes also, using a soft gaze, on a point about 5 feet ahead of you on the floor. Keep your gaze there but gently, without fixing your focus. Locate your breathing in your abdomen. You can do this by pushing your breath all the way out on the exhale and then sending your awareness to the in-and-out taking of your breath. Do this for 10 or so breaths, until you've located your breathing. Then just breathe naturally, without trying to breathe in any special way, but being aware of your breathing as it goes in and out of its own accord.

You might begin by sitting for 10 minutes a day, or 10 minutes twice a day, and then lengthen the time as you get used to the practice. Set a timer so that you don't need to watch the clock. It is more important to maintain a continuity of practice from day to day than to sit for longer periods of time. For example, sit for 10 minutes every day when you get up rather than sitting for 30 minutes on Monday and then not getting back to it until Thursday.

You will notice as you sit that your mind produces an endless stream of images, worries, plans, daydreams, and thoughts, both positive and negative. They race in, one after another. At the beginning stage, the realization of your mind's energy that spins out these random thoughts can be shocking and disagreeable. This is what the Buddhist's call "monkey mind" or "grasshopper mind"—for obvious reasons. But meditation trains the mind to regard this endless stream as a passing show, no one thought more important than another. When you find yourself getting caught up in your plans for the day, a pressing appointment, anxiety about your children, meal plans, vacation plans, or fantasies, just label this "thinking" and return your awareness to your breathing and to the present moment.

The point is to stay alert and relaxed, letting thoughts come and go. When you catch yourself getting caught up in one of them, simply label it "thinking," and return to your breathing. This will happen over and over in the course of 10 minutes. Just keep starting over, going back to the breathing and bringing yourself back to the present. Meditation is sometimes falsely looked at as a way to "clear your mind." You will not clear it, but you will learn to regard it in a different way—with equanimity.

PROFESSIONAL THERAPY

Much of what we've been talking about has to do with combating stress through our own efforts. But sometimes our problems become more than we can handle alone. That's when, blessedly, we can turn to professional institutions and people to help us. For example, we highly recommend twelve-step programs such as Alcoholics Anonymous and similar programs designed to help us kick bad habits and heal us of the shame that helped plunge us into the dependency in the first place. In a support group you can share your most painful feelings of shame, guilt, and stress without losing face. And listening to the moving and sometimes heroic stories of others helps put our own situation in perspective.

These days, support groups are available to almost everyone. Many of us have found that being in a protected space where we can laugh freely, and cry, is in itself good medicine. It is also, for people who have allowed shame and powerlessness to isolate them, the beginning of a return to the social world.

Finally, when all else fails, there is therapy. Your doctor or your minister should be able to recommend to you a counselor who can provide the help you need. Sometimes a few sessions do the job, by shifting our focus that half inch necessary to bring us back to positive life. Sometimes it takes longer. Sometimes the counseling is sufficient. Sometimes it's necessary to get a prescription for one of the many effective antidepressants or stress relievers available these days. Therapy is there for you. It's a tool for your benefit. Don't hesitate to use it to your advantage.

Our basic theme is simple, and we'll repeat it one more time to be sure that it's clear: No one has to be driven over the edge of despair by stress. Resources are available to help us find our way back to a productive and loving life.

No one has to be driven over the edge of despair by stress. Resources are available to everyone to help us find our way back to productive and loving life.

Although we have suggested strategies for relieving stress that have worked for many people, we don't pretend to know all the answers and we don't wish to oversimplify the problem. Life is often unfair and being black in America is often stressful. "Living under the veil," as Dr. W. E. B. Dubois described it, is unfortunately a reality for many of us. At times, the stress of everyday life can seem more than we can bear. That is why we must hold in mind not only the strategies we've listed in this chapter but also that old but powerful black saying: "The day we did things right was the day we stood up to fight. Keep your eyes on the prize and hold on."

Chapter 10

CORONARY ARTERY DISEASE AND EXERCISE

ELIZABETH TURNER, at fifty, had her working life where she wanted it. Five years earlier she'd quit her job and launched an interior decorating business. Now she had four people working with her and they were getting more work than they could handle. But as good as her work life was going, she couldn't say much for her love life. Her husband had left her three years earlier for another woman—younger, thinner, and, in her husband's eyes, at least, prettier. Elizabeth's self-esteem had been shattered. To make matters worse, the divorce hadn't gone as she wanted. Despite the fact that her job was at least as demanding as her ex's, she had full-time responsibility for the children and a lot less financial help from him than she felt entitled to.

On Tuesday morning, everything seemed to be coming to a head. She was gulping coffee and a cheese danish, getting ready to run off to the class she was taking three mornings a week. She was working toward her MBA degree and wondering if she could really keep up this juggling act—the kids, the job, and school. Out of the corner of her eye she'd been watching on TV a group of disgustingly fit young women go through their aerobic routine. "Why is it they never show any women but thin ones?" she asked herself. She wasn't fat, but she had put on some weight during the bad days of the marriage, and a bit more during the stress and loneliness of the divorce and its aftermath.

She kept watching. The women looked good, she had to admit, and they seemed to be having a good time, bouncing up and down to Janet Jackson's "Rhythm Nation." She remembered when she'd looked like that, when she'd danced like that and felt like that, that sweet energy and health running through her like a strong river. "God, what I wouldn't give to be young again!"

Then she sighed. "You grow up, girl—you can't turn back that big clock. Anyway, they've got men taking care of them and they're not juggling all the stuff I do. Yeah, exercise. If I tried to jog around here, they'd have me in the ER in no time for asphyxiation. No use feeling sorry for myself. I can still turn a few heads, and anyway, the life I lead, where would I find time for exercise even if I wanted to?" She gulped down the last of her coffee and danish and headed for the door.

Elizabeth Turner does not know that exercise is vital for the heart—a necessity, not a luxury. No way around that. It doesn't matter what your genetic history is or whether you're heart is strong or weak. It doesn't matter how healthy you may feel. Exercise is essential for the heart. And, while it's always easy

Exercise is vital for the heart—a necessity, not a luxury.

to think you just don't have time for another thing, this is one thing you can't afford to avoid.

Remember, the heart is a muscle—*the* muscle. When you don't use your arms, your biceps and forearms get flabby. When you don't use your legs, they get flabby. And so it is with the heart. "But my heart's beating. Isn't that all the exercise it needs?" No, it isn't. You might as well say that because you can lift a cup to your lips your arm muscles are working. Muscles, including the heart, follow the maxim, "Grow or die." They want to be used as vigorously as your age and condition allows. For your heart to be healthy, you must work it. And that means exercise, even if the exercise is simply half an hour of brisk walking once or twice a day.

*Remember, the heart is a muscle—*the muscle*, it's fair to say. When you don't use your arms, your biceps and forearms get flabby. When you don't use your legs, they do too. And so it is with the heart.*

What about those athletes and wannabes who die running or playing games when they'd have done better to stay home in bed or in front of the TV? Well, you can wiggle all you want. You can fool yourself all you want. But the fact of the matter is that to stay healthy, to reverse or prevent heart disease, or to recover from a heart attack, a proper exercise routine is the most important medicine you can take.

Americans in general don't exercise enough, but the problem is worse in the African American community. Studies suggest that nearly two thirds of African American men and a still greater number of African American women aren't active enough to stay healthy. For many of us, this inactivity leads to obesity. This is a special problem for African American women, nearly 40 percent of whom are overweight. You already know that fighting obesity isn't just a matter of vanity. Carrying extra weight means a greater likelihood of cholesterol buildup, and therefore of heart disease and heart attack. It can mean high blood pressure and diabetes.

Nearly two thirds of African American men and a still greater number of African American women aren't active enough to stay healthy.

Some researchers have suggested that the reason African American women are more likely than white women to be obese is that black women burn fewer calories when they are at rest than do white women. Others, such as Shiriki Kumanyiki, professor of epidemiology at Penn State College of Medicine, as cited in the *Health and Human Development Online Magazine,* attribute this difference to stress. And still others blame it on domestic arrangements (single mothers have no time to exercise) or socioeconomic factors (poor people can't go to health clubs and the neighborhoods aren't safe enough to allow jogging and other aerobic exercise). But the fact is that many of America's, and the world's, greatest athletes are African American—female athletes as well as male athletes. So it's obviously not impossible for African Americans to keep ourselves healthy and strong. Still, impossible or not, the data show that black Americans don't exercise as much as whites, and that this is one reason why heart disease and hypertension in the African American community are more common and, when incurred, more severe. (Remember, the death rate from heart disease is 40 percent higher for black men and 70 percent higher for black women than for their white counterparts.)

We don't mean to dismiss any of the explanations. We don't even dismiss the excuses. There are always lots of good reasons not to exercise. We wish only to establish what seems unarguable: that the reasons for exercising far outweigh most of the reasons against it. Exercise, by strengthening the heart muscle, makes heart disease less likely. But exercise also assures that, should you require a heart operation or other medical treatment, your chance of recovery will be far greater.

Speaking to you from my perspective as a heart surgeon, I find that some of my older patients—people in their seventies and eighties—do better after heart surgery than do people thirty and forty years their juniors. That's true, at least, when the older people have kept active, and when they've lived clean and healthy lives. Often, too, these older persons are less inclined to be overweight.

I hope we've made our case. Whether you have had a heart attack or have coronary artery disease or congestive heart failure, or you simply want to help prevent those problems from occurring, nothing will serve you better than a good and steady exercise program developed in cooperation with a doctor and perhaps a trainer. You need strong determination, which means promising yourself, when you start, that you will continue.

If you haven't been doing anything to get your body moving, you can make the promise to yourself: I will exercise for at least thirty minutes three times every week. A real aerobic exercise routine ought to be at least three times a week. If you take on only that minimal program of thirty minutes each session, you're giving only ninety minutes of your week to what is your best chance of long life and good health. To us, that looks like a better investment than anything you'll find on Wall Street.

While you won't believe it at first, you'll soon find the routine that felt like pulling teeth when you started becomes your favorite part of the week. You've all heard of those feel-good hormones called endorphins that exercise gets flowing. They're real, as everyone who follows a regular routine knows. So it's not just good health we're talking about here. It's literal, plain, old-fashioned feeling good. When you miss a day of exercise, your body will complain. If you're an older person, exercise will literally, honestly and truly, make you feel years younger. We know older people, and a few not so old, who, when they're forced to miss a week of exercise, can hardly get out of a chair, but when they're keeping at it regularly, are as lively as ever.

You've all heard of those feel-good hormones called endorphins that exercise gets flowing. They're real. So it's not just good health we're talking about here. It's literal, plain, old-fashioned feeling good.

Moderation here, as in all things, is the ticket. If you are elderly, or have been inactive, or have medical problems, you'll want to consult your doctor before beginning an exercise program. And, naturally, we don't want you exercising until you're breathless or experiencing heart pains. Nor do we want you walking around feeling sore from overexertion all the time. You're not training for a marathon or triathlon (though we know plenty of people who, without being superathletes, have done just that out of patience and persistence). No, we're recommending moderate exercise three times a week for thirty minutes each session. If you like to count, count calories. Burn 2,000 a week. That's a good counter's goal. You can do it on an exercise bike for forty-five minutes four times a week, or jogging on the treadmill or riding a stationary bicycle for thirty minutes three or four times a week, along with some vigorous walking on the off days.

Aerobic exercise, besides being perfect for your heart, is a better stress reliever than eating, smoking, drinking, or drugs. Each of the others involves cycles of dependency and craving. While taking your mind off the things you might be worried or angry about, exercise replaces negative feelings with a positive sense of well-being. So the greater the stress you're experiencing, the more important it is to exercise. Like meditation, exercise refreshes your mind, restores you, and helps you to face what had seemed overwhelming. So, let's review the core of the message. Moderate exercise

- Decreases blood pressure
- Raises good cholesterol (HDL)
- Lowers bad cholesterol (LDL)
- Lowers fat or triglyceride levels
- Helps burn body fat
- Helps relieve depression
- Builds confidence and self-esteem
- Encourages you to make other lifestyle changes
- Provides, with proper diet, an effective means of controlling noninsulin diabetes

And remember, when you exercise, do it for you—not for your partner.

Like meditation, exercise refreshes your mind, restores you, lets you face what had seemed overwhelming problems and, through the perspective and clarity that regular cleansing of your mind can provide, tackle challenges that had seemed impossible to meet.

EXERCISE PRECAUTIONS

Obviously, there are precautions to keep in mind. If you have had heart problems or a heart attack, no matter what your age, talk to your doctor before you begin to ensure that your heart can tolerate exercise. The same warning, of course, applies if you are recovering from bypass surgery, angioplasty, or stenting.

If you have had heart problems or a heart attack, no matter what your age, talk to your doctor before you begin to ensure that your heart can tolerate exercise.

Those over forty who haven't exercised in a long time should consult their doctor before starting an exercise program. And, of course, if you experience sudden shortness of breath or chest pains, stop exercising and get help. If it's extremely hot, avoid exercise outdoors or in a room that isn't air-conditioned and avoid outdoor exercise if it's extremely cold. Don't exercise when you're ill with a cold or flu, and don't exercise immediately after you eat, because it can cause cramps or nausea. Wait an hour or two, preferably two.

Keep in mind, too, that if you're beginning to exercise after a long layoff, you'll need to build yourself up. Maybe you used to be able to swim seventy-six laps without breathing heavily. But now you're fifty and a little out of shape and can only swim two without stopping. Swim two. After you've done that three times for a week, you'll feel ready to swim a lap or two more. That's the beauty of exercise. You get stronger and you can measure your progress. (Don't attempt to measure it at every session. Once a week is enough. That's when you can weigh yourself or gauge other progress.)

Maybe you once jogged five miles, but it's been a long time since you've walked more than three blocks. Start out with brisk walking. Feel your strength return. Before long, you may find yourself back to that five-mile jog. Moderation is the key.

Whatever exercise you're doing, spend a few minutes stretching and warming up before you begin. It will help you avoid injuries. By the same token, wear good, supporting shoes, comfortable clothing, and, if you're running or speed walking, avoid hard surfaces if at all possible. Many people jog in the streets these days, but if you're one of them, take reasonable care. It's easy to injure a foot or ankle on pavement.

Just as it is necessary to warm up, you also need to cool down when you've finished. That helps keep you from getting stiff and sore later. Cooling down is also beneficial because it allows your heart to return to its normal pace before you resume other activities. What this boils down to is that if you plan an hour of exercise, add fifteen minutes to it for warming up and cooling down.

GETTING STARTED

We're ready to go. You've set realistic goals for yourself, and you've vowed to make exercise a regular part of your routine, just like eating, showering, and sleeping. You're ready to tune in to your body. It will tell you if you're overdoing it; it will tell you when it's exhausted. Sometimes, to be sure, when you're just starting, it will lie a little. Like you, it's out of practice, and the first time you break into a brisk walk, or try to pick up a light weight, it will start complaining.

Learn to distinguish the heart's resistance from its real distress.

Learn to distinguish that resistance from real distress. In any case, once you have established your routine, the body gives up this resistance.

Remember: You aren't competing. When you first step into the gym, you may find yourself surrounded by lots of people who are in better shape than you. They aren't your concern. The simple trick about an exercise routine is that you begin where you are. If five-pound weights are all you can handle at the beginning, handle them. You'll be amazed that in a few weeks the ten-pounders will feel just right. You'll learn, after a while, that the weekly improvement you experience is all the competition you need. And even when you hit a plateau, the fact that you know you're healthier, and look better, and feel good, is quite enough.

Just as you need to be moderate in your goals, you can be moderate in your expenditure. These days, gyms can be fashion showcases. But all you need is a shirt and shorts, a pair of gym shoes and a pair of socks. Sure, you want the right shoes for what you're doing. But here too you can usually find bargains. Shop around. And don't spend a lot of money on exercise machines. If you belong to a gym, you'll find the machines there. If you don't, there's plenty of exercise you can do with minimal or no equipment.

In most neighborhoods there's a nearby community club or YMCA where you can work out regardless of your income. But if you are broke and don't have a free gym available in a neighboring school or social center, you can get along fine by buying a few weights and an inexpensive book that tells you what to do with them. If the streets of your neighborhood aren't fit for fast walking or jogging, go to a mall and walk around it three or four times. Or get on a bike or bus and go to a neighborhood that's safer.

When you're doing aerobic exercise—running, biking, swimming, or using a treadmill or stair climber—keep drinking water around to avoid dehydration. And use your mind along with your body. Many great athletes use mental imagery before they compete, fixing in their minds the actions they'll soon be performing. You too, before you start your exercise, should take a few deep breaths and bring to mind the specific action you are about to perform. If you're getting ready to run or begin some other aerobic exercise, imagine your proud finish. You'll find that such images can give you strength and courage, and can take your mind off the mere grinding aspect of exercise. It's a technique that works for champions. It can also work for you.

Use your mind along with your body. Many great athletes use mental imagery before they compete, fixing in their minds the actions they'll soon be performing.

Early morning and late night are good times for exercise. These are times when you can find an hour or two for yourself—though admittedly, if you're a working parent (single or not), that may require getting up a bit earlier or going to sleep a bit later. In the morning, an exercise routine will energize you for the day. In the evening, it will relax you and help you unload tension (though you may wish to avoid exercising just before bedtime, because the stimulation may make it harder for you to fall asleep.)

Okay? Let's get it on. Your goal is to burn 2,000 to 3,000 calories per week, at the rate of 300 to 500 calories per exercise period. Here's the menu:

CALORIE EXPENDITURE FOR ATHLETIC ACTIVITIES

These figures apply to a person weighing 150 pounds. Allow a 10 percent increase in caloric expenditure for every 15 pounds over 150, and a 10 percent decrease for every 15 pounds under 150.

Activity	**Calories Per Hour**
Aerobic dancing	280–700
Backpacking	350–770
Badminton (competitive singles)	480
Basketball	360–600
Bicycling	
(10 mph)	420
(11 mph)	480
(12 mph)	600
(13 mph)	660
Calisthenics (heavy)	600
Gardening, lifting, stooping, digging	500
Golf (pull-carry clubs)	280–490
Handball	660
Hiking	660
Horseback riding	210–560
Mowing (push mower)	450
Rope skipping, vigorous	800
Rowing machine	840

Calorie Expenditure for Athletic Activities, continued

Activity	**Calories Per Hour**
Running	
(5 mph)	600
(6 mph)	750
(7 mph)	870
(8 mph)	1,020
(9 mph)	1,130
(10 mph)	1,235
Shoveling (heavy)	660
Skating, ice or roller, rapid	700
Skiing, downhill	600
Skiing, cross-country	
(2.5 mph)	560
(4 mph)	600
(5 mph)	700
(8 mph)	1,020
Snowshoeing	490–980
Swimming (25–50 yd/min)	360–750
Tennis, singles	420–480
Tennis, doubles	300–360
Walking, level road,	
4 mph (fast)	420
up stairs	600–1,080
up hill (3.5 mph)	480–900
Wood chopping	560

CALORIES BURNED ACCORDING TO WEIGHT

Activity	100 lb.	150 lb.	200 lb.
Bicycling, 6 mph	160	240	312
Bicycling, 12 mph	270	410	534
Jogging, 7 mph	610	920	1,230
Jump roping	500	750	1,000
Running, 5.5 mph	440	660	962
Running, 10 mph	850	1,280	1,664
Swimming, 25 yd/min	185	275	358
Swimming, 50 yd/min	325	275	650
Tennis, singles	265	400	535
Walking, 2 mph	160	240	312
Walking, 3 mph	210	320	416
Walking, 4.5 mph	295	440	572

OUR FINAL INSTRUCTIONS

How do you know when you are exercising at the proper rate? Check your pulse. You'll have determined, with your doctor, the proper target rate. To find your pulse, the simplest method is to put your index and middle fingers on your radial artery, which you can feel pulsing just where the wrist merges with the forearm. Watching the second hand on a clock or your wristwatch,

How do you know when you are exercising at the proper rate? Check your pulse.

count the number of times your pulse beats in fifteen seconds, and multiply by four.

You can also take your pulse at the carotid artery in the neck by placing your index and middle fingers on the sternomastoid muscle. It's the one you feel when you turn your head to the side. Then count by the method described above. But don't press too hard. That can cause the heart to slow, or, if you have had carotid disease or a history of ministrokes, it may even cause a stroke. For that reason, check with your doctor before using this method—especially if you have diabetes or have had a stroke or previous brain damage.

Once again, a few warnings: Chest discomfort or tightness, or arm or neck pain during exercise, could be signs of angina.

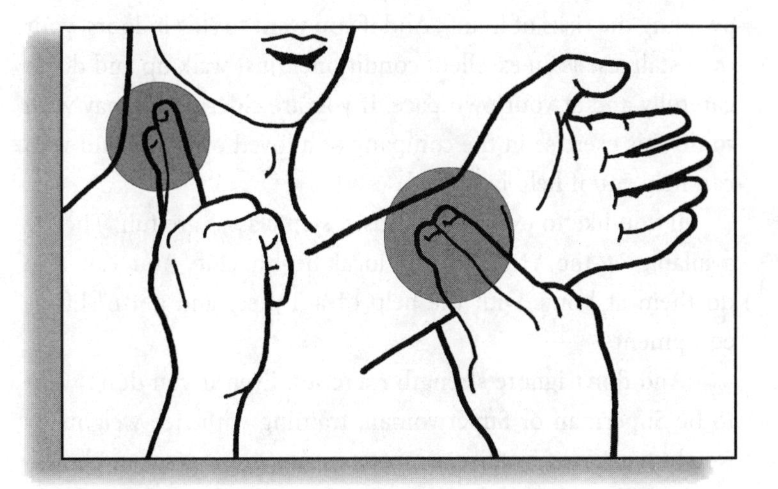

Check your heart rate by counting your pulse at the neck or wrist

Stop what you are doing and call for help or dial 911. Severe shortness of breath or excessive coughing while you're exercising also means you should stop. The same is true of bone or joint discomfort or severe muscle cramps or tendon soreness. Faintness, nausea, or vomiting during exercise means you should stop and see your doctor. The bottom line is listen to your body and obey what it tells you.

Choose the form of exercise that feels most comfortable. Get your friends involved—take walks with them in the morning at a mall, a park, or a schoolyard. Walk to work if you can, and always walk rather than drive when the distances allow. Take a walk during your lunch break to a bookstore or to a place where you can eat lunch and rest your mind at the same time.

Remember that aerobics don't necessarily mean running, nor do they require equipment. Fast walking or power walking are excellent exercises, giving most of the benefits of running, but avoiding the risks of injury. And if you want to stay indoors, your own staircase is an excellent conditioner. Just walk up and down carefully and at your own pace. If you are elderly, you may wish to do this exercise in the company of a loved one or friend who can help you if help is needed.

If you like to exercise to music, step classes are fun. They're available at the YMCA, your local health club. You can also do them at home with the help of a TV set and a 4-6" lift as equipment.

And don't ignore strength exercises. Even if you don't want to be Superman or Superwoman, training with free weights or weight machines, just like aerobic exercise, improves your cholesterol profile, helps control your weight, and helps control conditions such as diabetes. Because such exercises also enhance flexibility and balance, they help you live with degenerative diseases like arthritis. Weight training isn't reserved for men. Because women often suffer muscle atrophy, it is also most beneficial to them.

In working with weights, especially free weights, have an instructor nearby, especially when you begin. And remember that it's far better to go for multiple repetitions at a comfortable weight than to try to impress people by pushing weights far too heavy for you. Your aim is to improve your muscle tone and strength, but not, as power lifters do, to go for bulk.

The world is your gym. You don't need riches or power to join. Your own body, just as it is, is the only ticket required for admission.

Before we close this part of the discussion, we want to say a few words about exercising when you suffer from a disease that weakens you or in some other way prevents you from performing fully. Arthritis is one such disease. A degenerative joint disease, it's often associated with pain, and those who suffer from it can't handle weights without making that pain worse. For them, the most popular exercise is swimming. But bicycling is also a good sport for sufferers from arthritis, unless knee pain prevents it.

Patients with diabetes can also benefit from exercise. It helps lower the blood sugar, and in some cases even allows the patient to go off medication or insulin. Walking is an excellent exercise for diabetics. Remember that the appropriate footwear is important, to help protect the feet and legs from injury caused by the poor blood flow that accompanies diabetes.

Patients recovering from heart surgery or a heart attack will do supervised exercise as part of their cardiac rehab program.

Once that's done, with their doctor's approval, they will return to normal life—which means normal exercise.

Finally, if your cholesterol or triglyceride levels are abnormally high, exercise will decrease bad cholesterol (LDL) and triglyceride levels. And aerobic exercise increases good cholesterol.

Chapter 11

THE AFRICAN AMERICAN WOMAN AND HEART DISEASE

> You hear about men having heart attacks. . .; many women are the caretakers for those men, but they don't know that heart attacks and heart disease are permanent among women. I love the theme "Take wellness to heart." Women take so many things—we take our responsibility of being wives, being daughters, being members of the community—but not frequently, not seriously enough, do we take our own wellness to heart.
>
> —*Maya Angelou*

THE DAY THAT Christy's body sent her bad news ought to have been one of the best days of her life. She had just gotten the promotion she'd long aimed for: Now she was the first African American woman ever to be appointed senior vice president at a major telecommunications company in Chicago. She had weathered many storms to get there and also managed, with the help of intelligence, quick wit, and a sense of humor, to keep her children and her husband happy. She had experienced many minor and some major episodes of sexism and racism that threatened to derail her, and she often had to move fast and think on her feet. She had fought some big battles, and avoided the ones that seemed avoidable. She had paid costs—not exercising regularly, letting the intensity of the chase drive her back to cigarettes, getting less rest than she needed, and never being quite able to relax. And she'd sometimes known the terrible isolation and depression of being the only African American woman at board meetings. Often, she found herself repeating what her grandmother had taught her: "Keep your eye on the prize and hold on." Now, she thought, she was where she had wanted to be for so long. Time to enjoy it and know some inner peace.

That's when her body sent its message: a heaviness in her chest and a wave of indigestion, along with a wave of fatigue. Actually, she'd had these sensations off and on for nearly a year now, but this time, as she drove along Lake Shore Drive on her way to her home in Hyde Park, she couldn't dismiss them as merely the stress of climbing toward her goal. She'd read in the *Essence* health columns that African American women were 70 percent more likely than white women to die if they suffered a heart attack. She knew that her risks increased as she got older, and that as she approached menopause the risks were especially strong, because the beneficial effects of estrogen on the heart lessen. That was the message her body sent her now, in this wonderful moment of her life, as she drove home to share with her family the joy she felt: She feared that she was suffering the symptoms of a heart problem.

Still, once home, she masked her fear. She checked in with the kids, hugged them, and oversaw their homework for a while.

When Frank came home, she told him the good news. Together, they celebrated over a couple of glasses of wine. Then, in the midst of love and shared happiness, she felt herself nodding off. She roused herself, then, once again, slipped down into darkness. . . .

She could hear Frank telling the 911 operator that his wife had had a heart attack—that she wasn't breathing and he feared she was dead. The children were around her as he spoke, hugging her and shaking her and calling her name. She was telling Frank it was all right, she was all right. She was telling the children the same thing, not to worry. But Frank and the children didn't seem to hear her. She was very frightened and prayed that this was all a bad dream.

It had to be a dream. She couldn't lose all this now—her family, the comfort she and Frank had built around them, the fruit of her enormous investment of self in her family and in her work. She saw it all slipping away. She saw the life that she'd help make vanish like smoke. She saw Frank and the children and her friends praying at her graveside, and she could hear them sobbing over her.

It was the sound of the children's sobbing that finally woke her. But when she woke, no one was sobbing. There they were, the people she most loved, the girls still at their homework at one end of the room, Frank smiling as she woke. When he saw the tears in her eyes, she had to explain her dream. "It was so terrible, baby, to lose you, to lose them, to lose everything. It was so real. And you know, it was real. That dream came from somewhere to tell me something. That dream said, "Stop running long enough to take care of yourself, or you're going to end up just being part of a percentage."

Christy's story had a happy ending. The dream was just a dream. She began to build into her busy day periods when she'd empty herself of busyness and stress. She started giving more attention to her exercise and diet. Of course, she quit smoking, this time for good. And before long, over another glass of wine, she was able to tell Frank: "You know, baby, I don't feel as if I'm going to end up part of that percentage after all." But every day women have Christy's bad dream, only to find that it isn't a dream at all. Half a million women die each year of cardiovascular disease—more than die of the next sixteen causes of death combined.

> Black women have the highest death rate of heart disease and develop it at an earlier age than any other population in the United States.
>
> *Ann L. Taylor, M.D.*
> *Case Western Reserve University, Cleveland*

There are a lot of misconceptions about women and heart disease:

- Cardiovascular disease is something that just happens to men. On the contrary, since the mid-Eighties, according to the American Heart Association, it has killed more women than men.
- Breast cancer is the major cause of death in women. Although surveys find that women are more afraid of breast cancer than of cardiovascular disease, breast cancer kills one in twenty-seven of those diagnosed; cardiovascular disease kills one in two.
- Coronary symptoms like angina and heart attacks are the same whether you are a man or a woman. In fact, the

symptoms often present themselves differently in women, which is explained later in this chapter.

You already know the most frightening fact of all: that African American women who suffer a heart attack are one and a half times more likely to die from it than white women. You can blame this fact on discrimination, but that would be only half true. African American women are more likely than white woman to suffer the major risk factors, which are high cholesterol, lack of exercise, diabetes, smoking, and being overweight.

Although 2.5 million women are hospitalized each year for heart disease or stroke and, sadly, 500,000 of these women die of those causes, little has been written about women and heart disease. (Twenty-five times more men than women have been studied in the area of heart disease.) Though sexism may be partly to blame here, and other explanations have been offered, the reason for the discrepancy is unclear. But whatever the cause, here is a case where not only the lay community but the medical community as well are often underinformed and misinformed.

DANGERS FOR WOMEN

According to some studies,[1] women between the ages of 35-64 years have a 30-45 percent chance of sudden death or dying after one year after a heart attack. Men in the same age bracket have a 10-16% chance of death suddenly or after one year. Naturally, the statistics are worse for older patients. When we add the fact that African American women are 70 percent more likely than white

---

1 Linda Ojeda, Ph.D. *Her Healthy Heart* (Hunter House, 1998), pp. 11-13.

> *When women reach the 65-70 age bracket they have about the same chance as men of developing heart disease.*

women to die of a heart attack, we have to wonder why the literature tends to suggest that coronary artery disease is a white man's problem.

We've mentioned some of the risk factors that make women in general and African American women in particular susceptible to heart disease. But there are also diagnostic and physiological reasons that make the death rates for women in general worse than those for men. Diagnosis of heart disease in women is often made later because doctors, and women themselves, are more likely to write off symptoms of chest pain and chest pressure as indigestion or stress or panic.

It's also true that, because women's arteries are smaller, there is a greater risk of blockage and decreased blood flow. Worse, because the arteries are smaller, remedial treatments such as angioplasty and coronary bypass grafting are often more difficult.

Finally, women are likely to experience coronary artery disease later in life than men. While they are still menstruating, estrogen helps protect the heart. It does this by preventing a plaque buildup by increasing the supply of good cholesterol and decreasing the supply of bad cholesterol. Estrogen may also open up (dilate) the blood vessels that feed blood to the heart—though this possibility is speculative.

Because these estrogen-related benefits aren't afforded to the postmenopausal woman, sometime between the mid-40s and early 50s a woman's risk of suffering coronary disease begins to climb and to approach a man's risk level. (Some doctors recommend estrogen replacement therapy as a remedy for this problem, but the studies on this subject are still inconclusive.) When women reach the 65-70 age bracket, they have about the same chance as men of developing heart disease. (Some studies suggest that men are susceptible earlier because at the end of puberty their high-density lipoproteins [HDL] decline dramatically.)

Diabetes

Diabetes, a condition in which the blood glucose level is high, is especially dangerous for women. Diabetics are especially susceptible to high blood pressure, cardiovascular disease and strokes. To make matters still worse, diabetics often have high cholesterol and thus increase their risk of heart disease even more. Fortunately, diabetes can be treated. But, even treated, diabetes increases the risk of stroke.

Obesity

One third of American women are overweight. Forty percent of African American women are overweight. Obesity not only increases the risk of heart disease but it also makes treatment, such as angioplasty or surgery, more difficult and their outcomes more problematic. Overweight patients are more likely to have respiratory problems and to have blood clots after heart surgery as well.

American women are overweight—one third of them. African American women are overweight—one half of them.

There are psychological burdens of obesity, which can also weigh heavily on a woman's health. Extremely overweight people tend to be depressed. Society is often cruel to them and they easily become isolated. That isolation, in turn, can make it less likely that they will seek medical help. Often, lack of self-esteem makes an overweight person less likely to take care of herself and therefore unwilling to turn to a doctor.

To disregard obesity is, in Maya Angelou's words, to not "take wellness to heart." In most cases, the tendency toward obesity can, with your goodwill and hard work and your doctor's help, be reversed.

Smoking

Cigarette smoking is even more dangerous to women than to men. The direct threat it poses to women is that it decreases the power of estrogen to protect the heart. According to the Framingham Heart Study, a woman who smokes cigarettes is at least twice and perhaps as much as six times more likely to have a heart attack than a woman who doesn't.[2] Admittedly, that's a wide range—but even the lower figure ought to be enough to convince you not to smoke.

Cigarette smoking is even more dangerous to women than to men. The direct threat it poses to women is that it decreases the power of estrogen to protect your heart.

To make matters more complicated and worse, the combination of smoking and oral contraceptives is especially lethal: It makes the likelihood of suffering a heart attack forty times as great, and of

2 For the Framingham study, see http://www.nhlbi.nih.gov/about/framingham/design/htm

suffering a stroke twenty times as great. We don't have to tell you that those are very bad numbers.

Unfortunately, oral contraceptives in themselves are a risk factor, because they decrease the protective effect of good cholesterol. Add smoking to this and you have a deadly cocktail.

Women, like men, often fear that if they stop smoking they will gain weight. Our only answer is that if you are on oral contraceptives, exercise and a better diet will help keep weight in line with far better results and much less risk. The trouble with the nicotine diet is that it's likely to kill you.

The combination of smoking and oral contraceptives is especially lethal.

High Blood Pressure

High blood pressure (hypertension) affects at least one in four African Americans. In at least ten percent of these cases it causes an enlarged heart, which is called left ventricular hypertrophy. That condition is often the first sign of heart disease and it is often irreversible. It's a condition that can cause sudden death. For many black women there's no second chance: The first sign of a heart problem can be a massive heart attack and sudden death.

Chronic Stress

Stress comes in many disguises and there's plenty of it to go around. Women often carry their burdens in relative isolation. Isolation, we know, can bring depression, and the two in combination can add up to deadly chronic stress.

Women often define themselves as caretakers. But in fulfilling that role, they risk leaving nothing for themselves. This problem is compounded by job stress. Many women are employees, wives, mothers, housekeepers and cooks, community servants, daughters who care for aging parents, and so on. They are involved in an all-consuming juggling act.

If this situation is typical for the middle-class woman, it can be even worse for the poor. Less education usually means lower-paying jobs. In addition, there is an increased sense of powerlessness. Often, women feel the stress of a bad marriage more than men do.

Finally, as we've seen, racism compounds these problems. Although difficult to measure, it's likely to be at least as bad for your health as smoking. We believe that if discrimination could be eliminated, the rate of heart disease in the African American community would drop dramatically.

We are left not with the prospect of reducing the causes of stress but with the need to control it—by treating our bodies right. We're not saying any of this is easy. We're just saying it's essential if you are to take your wellness to heart.

SYMPTOMS OF CORONARY DISEASE AND STRESS IN WOMEN

The warning signs for coronary disease are somewhat different in women than in men, and this, as we've said, is one reason why diagnosis for women sometimes comes late or not at all. Women's symptoms tend to be less dramatic and more heavily masked, easy to mistake for indigestion, fatigue, stress, or panic. The symptoms express themselves as:

- Uncomfortable pressure, fullness, squeezing, or pain in the center of the chest that lasts for more than a few minutes

- Light-headedness
- Fainting
- Sweating
- Nausea
- Shortness of breath
- Chronic fatigue

Remember that not all these symptoms occur in a particular attack every time. Sometimes the symptoms go away and return. But if some occur, the American Heart Association recommends—and we obviously agree—that you should get help fast. If you notice one or more of these signs in yourself or another person, call your emergency medical service (911 in most areas). The person needs to go to a hospital right away!

We again remind you that the patient will get the most prompt and efficient care if he or she is brought by ambulance to the hospital. Only if you are told that the ambulance can't come in a reasonable amount of time should you attempt to take your loved one to the hospital yourself.

Similarly, if you notice one of more of the following signs of stroke, call your emergency medical service immediately:

- Sudden weakness or numbness in the face, arm, or leg on one side of the body.
- Sudden dimness or loss of vision, particularly in one eye.
- Sudden loss of speech or trouble talking or understanding speech.
- Sudden severe headaches with no known or apparent cause.

- Sudden unexplained dizziness, unsteadiness, or falling, especially along with any of the other symptoms listed here.

Some of these symptoms may certainly prove to be signs of less serious problems such as indigestion or hyperventilation; others may in fact be the passing signs of temporary stress. But because women's symptoms have so often been fatally dismissed, it's best to be cautious. The Framingham study shows that nearly 33 percent of women's heart attacks aren't detected at the time they take place. The men's figure is much lower.[3] Further, according to a later study,[4] in sixty percent of the women's cases cardiac arrest was the first sign of heart disease that the patient experienced. Don't let yourself or a loved one be among that group. These figures can be changed in part by your knowing and listening to the signs, knowing the risk factors for coronary artery disease, and getting regular check ups. Above all, when in doubt, see your doctor. It is far better to seek treatment that proves unnecessary than not to seek it at all.

DIAGNOSIS AND TREATMENT

This section explains things that may not surprise us but that ought to shock us all. Men are more likely to get treatment for

---

3 See: Kannel, W. 1986. "Silent Myocardial Ischemia and Infarction: Insights from the Framingham Study," *Cardiology Clinics* 4 (4): 583-591.

4 Albert, C.B. McGovern, et al., in their 1996 study on "Sex Differences in Cardiac Arrest Survivors" *(Circulation* 93 [6]: 1170-1176.

heart disease than women; white women are more likely to get treatment than black women; poor people are less likely to get treatment than people who aren't poor. It doesn't have to be this way. We want to document it first and then talk about what you can do to change it.

A study of over 80,000 patients hospitalized for coronary disease[5] came to these sad conclusions:

- In cases of heart disease, men are more likely than women to be accurately diagnosed, to receive treatment, and to survive coronary bypass surgery than women. (See the rest of this list for details.)
- Traditional diagnostic tests for heart disease—namely, electrocardiograms (EKGs) or thallium tests—are less precise in defining coronary heart disease among women than among men.
- In the emergency room, after a heart attack, men are more likely than women to receive medications that dissolve clots (thrombolytic agents). This is in part because women are more likely to react to such medicines with greater complications such as internal bleeding.
- Men with heart disease are roughly 25 percent more likely to receive heart catheterization and 45 percent more likely to have bypass surgery or balloon angioplasty than women.

---

5 Ayanian, J. and A. Epstein. 1991. "Difference in Use of Procedures Between Men and Women Hospitalized for Coronary Heart Disease," *New England Journal of Medicine* 325 (4): 221-225.

Wayne Giles, M.D., of the University of Alabama at Birmingham,[6] has found that there are dramatic sexual and racial differences in the diagnosis and treatment of coronary disease. An African American is less likely than a white American to get coronary artery surgery, cardiac catheterization, or a stent. That difference holds even after factors such as insurance, the age of the patient, hospital admission, and hospital transfer are taken into account.

The situation outlined by Giles's study invites us to look for reasons. Most studies suggest that racism, access to care, and poverty account for the fact that, once they show symptoms of coronary disease, blacks are less likely than whites to receive diagnosis and treatment. A study by Mark B. Wenneker, M.D., and Arnold M. Epstine, M.D.[7] suggests that this difference in diagnosis and treatment may stem from a "stronger tendency [on the part of African Americans] to refuse high-tech options." Adrian Ostfeld agrees that "African Americans are less likely to agree to such procedures," and that that this "may reflect a continuing distrust by some African Americans of the medical establishment."

---

6 Wayne H. Giles, M.D., et al, "Race and Sex Differences in Rates of Invasive Cardiac Procedures in U.S. Hospitals," *Archives of Internal Medicine,* 1995. Other studies on racial differences in treatment include David M. Carlisle, M.D. et al, "Racial and Ethnic Differences in the Use of Invasive Cardiac Procedures Among Cardiac Patients in Los Angeles County, 1986-1988," *American Journal of Public Health,* March 1995 Vol. 85, No.3, p. 352-356; and Marianne Laouri, Ph.D. et al, "Underuse of Coronary Revascularization Procedures: Application of a Clinical Method," *Journal of American College of Cardiology.* 1997 29: 891-7.

7 Cited Barry Zaret, et al., *Yale University School of Medicine Heart Book (William Morrow, 1992),* p. 279.

Whatever the reason, the essential point is that there is a difference in the diagnosis and treatment of blacks and whites with coronary disease. Knowledge of this fact, along with a clear understanding of what should happen, will help eliminate the difference and decrease the overall death rate for black men and women who suffer heart disease. It's our hope that this book will play a part in that change.

TAKING YOUR WELLNESS TO HEART

If you are an African American woman, the threat of coronary artery disease and even death is very real. But taking control of your own life, rethinking your values in light of this threat can improve your chances greatly. You don't need to wait, as Christy did, for a bad dream from which you may or may not awake. Our aim here has been to awaken you before that sleep grows too deep. Make a solid commitment today to protect your heart and make the changes in your life that commitment requires.

1. *Gain knowledge.* A coronary patient armed with knowledge has better chances than one who isn't. Better yet, make the required changes before you become that patient.

2. *Ask questions and expect answers.* Ask your doctor to talk to you in a way you can understand. Have the confidence, self-respect, and commitment to your own health and to your loved ones to insist on a thorough understanding of what's going on. If the doctors fail to use tests that you believe are appropriate, find out why.

The American Heart Association recommends that you copy these questions and take them to your doctor on your next checkup:

- What are my risk factors for heart disease?
- Am I at risk for stroke?
- What are the warning signs or symptoms of heart disease and stroke?
- What should I know about the effects of menopause on my health?
- Do I need to lose or gain weight for my optimal health?
- What is a healthful eating plan for me?
- What kind of physical activity is right for me?
- What is my blood pressure? Is it healthy for my age?
- What is my cholesterol level and is it at a healthy level?
- Based on my personal history and risk factors, what can I do to lower my risk of heart disease and stroke? (Women who smoke should ask for assistance in quitting.)

You'll have learned the answers to some of these questions from this book. But it's not a bad idea to ask them anyway. They will let your doctor know that you are a woman ready to take her wellness to heart, and you'll therefore command his or her best attention and respect. If your doctor doesn't answer the questions to your satisfaction, talk to a second doctor or seek out the information yourself. The internet is an excellent source of medical information. The librarian at your local library or the hospital librarian will be glad to get you started if you need guidance. You can't afford to be ignorant about matters of the heart.

3. ***Know the risk factors specific to women and to African Americans in general.*** Meet them directly and conquer them. If you have high blood pressure, take your medication. Take your insulin if you are diabetic. Whether or not you are overweight, exercise regularly and watch what you eat. If you are overweight, diet as well. Use the chapters on nutrition and the appendix on healthy cooking methods as your guide.

   And—we'll say it again—exercise regularly. Take at least as much pride in caring for your body as you do in caring for your hair or your makeup or your clothes. Exercise is a lifelong commitment, and you need to do it three times a week. Exercise relieves stress and makes your heart strong. There's nothing better you can do for yourself.

4. ***Avoid stress when you can, and manage it when you can't avoid it.*** Remember that you have evolved from generations and generations of women who were successful against great odds, who met their challenges with courage and faith. Make yourself one of them.

5. ***Remain or become part of a social group.*** Regular contact with people you share interests and values with is as good for your heart as it is for your soul.

6. ***Equally important, don't be too busy yourself and don't let the other people in your family be too busy to share feelings, ideas, and concerns.*** Hold family meetings once or twice a week and insist that all family members attend. Stress grows out of the pains and frustrations that we don't get a chance, or don't take a chance, to articulate. Give everyone in your family, yourself included, a chance to do that.

7. ***Keep a journal.*** It's a way to release your thoughts and emotions. Besides, you'll be surprised by what an interesting person you turn out to be. Writing a journal is an excellent method of stress management. But don't forget to reread your writing.

8. ***No matter how busy you are, take regular time out for yourself each day.*** Maybe it's the first thing you do when you get up, or the last thing before going to sleep. But take it. You owe it to yourself. At such times you may want to review the past day or plan the next day. Also, leave yourself fifteen or twenty minutes a day simply to meditate or pray or just find quiet time. You'll be surprised to see the benefits that come from giving yourself this gift of peaceful calm and quiet.

Chapter 12

THE FACTS ABOUT DIET AND LIFESTYLE

KENYA WAS GOING HOME, and though she didn't expect a parade, she thought that an astronaut returning to earth from a moon shot must feel a lot like she felt. She'd graduated from Harvard Medical School, one of eleven African Americans of the twenty who had started out in her class. Not only was she the first in her family to go to college but she was the first in her neighborhood to get a college degree, let alone a medical degree. She had also been one of the best premedical students to graduate from Howard University. No, the astronauts didn't have anything on her—she'd been to the moon, and now she was coming back, to Indianapolis, her hometown, to start her residency in the field of internal medicine, at University Hospital.

On the plane, Kenya lounged in the first-class seat she'd given herself as a reward, thinking of the sleepless nights behind her, the sleepless nights to come, the utter concentration Howard and

Harvard had demanded of her, and the even more complete self-surrender she'd be making during her residency. But the knowledge that she had more than measured up to past challenges, and the certainty that she had to be up to those to come, made her feel a little giddy. As she got off the plane in Indianapolis and headed for the car rental, the astronaut fantasy returned, and for a moment she found herself walking with the kind of clumsy confidence of a woman in a space suit.

The home planet had changed some, she thought. People moved a little slower and talked a little slower than they did on the moon. But she knew she could get used to that again. It hadn't been so easy to adjust to that moon pace anyway.

It took her a while to get to her parents' new neighborhood in the suburb. To see block after block of green lawns and fresh paint, good roofs and clean sidewalks, made her heart glad. It was Saturday and the people looked so pretty and peaceful, walking their dogs, jogging, carefree and at ease. They came out of the health food store a few blocks from her parents' house drinking spring water and fruit juices, dressed for bicycling or jogging, looking like they spent time in the gym. Well-dressed kids walked along holding their parents' hands.

When Kenya stopped at the supermarket a block later to find a cake for her mother's birthday, she was dazzled by a produce department that stretched the length of the store, stocked with fruits and vegetables that looked like they'd just come from the tree or the ground. At the butcher's counter she found only fine cuts of fresh, lean meat, and next to it, a display of fresh fish as good as any she'd seen in Washington or Cambridge. It comforted her to think that this was the store where her parents shopped.

It was three in the afternoon when she'd found her cake—the cake in a garden of perfect cakes: "Too early to go to my folks' house," she thought. "They said they wouldn't be back until four." So she drove out to the old neighborhood that she hadn't visited since her parents left it three years ago. As she drove, the houses got smaller and dingier. The yards shrank too, and instead of spreading lawns and brilliant flowers, there was a lot of bare dirt, only here and there yards that looked like they'd got much recent attention. There were clusters of people hanging out on the street corners, but she no longer saw joggers. "Yeah," she remembered, "life itself is often all the exercise people can handle back in the 'hood."

Close to her old home she parked the car and began to walk. Nobody actually looked at her, but she could feel the old pressures, whiffs of fear, the sense that she was overdressed now, that she'd become a foreigner. "C'mon girl, you gotta snap out of this," she told herself. "These are your streets; these are your people. Don't forget where you came from."

She felt relieved when she saw the grocery store she'd known as a kid, the window still splashed with handwritten signs announcing today's specials. But when she went in, the relief faded. No sign of Mr. and Mrs. Brown, who used to run the store. Now a surly middle-aged white man was behind the counter, and he didn't look especially happy to see her.

"How're you doing?" Kenya said. "You know, I grew up in this store. This is where we used to get our candy and soda pop after school when I was a kid. Mind if I look around for old time's sake?"

He grunted something that didn't sound reassuring, but she looked around anyway. The meat looked gray, and there wasn't much selection—ribs, fatback, old-looking chicken, some chitlings, a few sad-looking pork chops. At the fish display, through the fly specks, she could make out nothing but catfish and perch, and they looked like they hadn't seen the water in a long time. There were few vegetables, and what there was was limp and faded.

Kenya bought herself a pack of chewing gum on the way out, though she hadn't chewed gum in years. Back on the street she unwrapped a piece. It tasted as stale as the fish looked, and as she chewed, she felt for a minute as if she were about to cry. A block or two down the street, at a major intersection, she saw a string of fast-food restaurants. After leaving that sad little grocery store, she saw how easy it would be to slip into the fast-food habit. "It's as if they were pushing one more kind of junk at us," Kenya said to herself.

As if to confirm the thought, the billboard that loomed over the next intersection featured a black couple in their 30s, well dressed and smug-looking, the woman looking at the man with an admiring smile. The man was good-looking, of course, and he held a cigarette in one hand and a glass of cognac in the other. Across the street from the billboard was a liquor store, so crowded that Kenya couldn't see past the front door.

By this time, Kenya's anger had soured the fine mood she'd arrived with. Now everything she saw seemed part of a single message. She passed good-looking girls in the street, but she couldn't help seeing that many of them were overweight. And as she passed the front porches of some of the houses, smells of barbecue filled the air. Childhood memories came back in a rush—happy uncles and aunts, her own sisters and brothers and cousins around her, the comfort and happiness of being with family. And people putting down slabs of ribs, great chunks of chicken smothered in hot sauce, hamburgers, hot dogs, corn smothered in real butter, great slabs of pie—wonderful food, but also one of the big reasons why so many African Americans she knew suffered from heart disease, and why their mortality rate was so high.

That night, while in her parents' backyard, neighbors and relatives gathered to celebrate her mother's birthday, Kenya felt the good old feeling again. She was home with her people. She was where she belonged. But as she watched the others eat, and while she put down her own share of juicy and delicious ribs, she knew she was caught in a struggle that would go on for a long time. It was wonderful to eat this food. It warmed her soul. But it was party food, celebration food, and it needed to be eaten in moderation. She felt she had a gospel to preach, about loving the body God gave you, about the good health that we owed to ourselves and to each other. But how could she say it? Everything in the culture seemed to be lined up against her.

Let's leave Kenya for a minute and repeat a few facts:

- Coronary artery disease is the number one killer of African American women and men.
- In 1995, heart disease mortality was 40 percent higher for African Americans than for whites.[1]

---

1 Taylor Jr., M.D. Herman et al, "Long-Term Survival of African American in the Coronary Artery Surgery Study," *Journal of American College of Cardiology* 1997; 29: 358-64; Roig M.D., Eulalia "In Hospital Mortality Rates from Acute Myocardial Infarction by Race in U.S. Hospitals: Finding from the National Hospital Discharge Survey," *Circulation* (1987)76, No. 2, 280-288.

- From 1988 to 1994, 35 percent of black males ages 20 to 74 had hypertension compared with 25 percent of white men in the same age group.
- According to a Chicago Heart Association survey, the rate of obesity among African Americans is higher than it is among whites, and the risk of early coronary artery disease and death is also higher.
- Among adult women, the age-adjusted prevalence of obesity continues to be higher for African American women (40 percent) than for white women.
- According to surveys by Cardia and Minnesota Heart, African American women exercise less, and, in general, have lower levels of physical activity than white women.
- More than one third of both nonfatal and fatal heart attacks among African American women may be attributed to obesity.[2]

It all adds up to a single, clear message. Maybe we can't cure poverty. Maybe we can't cure the racism that still plagues our country. But as African Americans we can do much more toward curing ourselves from the disease that afflicts us more than others. We can take matters into our own hands by giving our hearts the nurture they require to feed our lives with strength and vitality.

African Americans can do much more toward curing ourselves from the disease that afflicts us.

2 See Sheree Crute, ed.,*Health and Healing for African Americans* (Bantam Books, 1998) p. 30.

Let's begin with the hardest part of the problem. It won't surprise you to learn, according to recent studies, that black men with high blood pressure suffered a worsening of that condition because of steady emotional stress brought on by racial discrimination.[3] Other studies show that unemployment and other economic insecurity also contribute to the risk and severity of heart disease. So, of course, does chronic emotional distress, accompanied by feelings of anxiety, paranoia, exhaustion, and hostility—a stress that, as we all know, is part of a black person's legacy in America.

It's precisely because these incurable conditions exist that some African Americans neglect to take responsibility for their health. "You gotta be kidding me," they might say. "I'm supposed to worry about my blood pressure when every time I go out the door I walk into a world that has nothing better to do than set it soaring? Let me at least eat and drink as I please, and take my pleasures where I find them."

There's no easy answer to that argument. But there is a hard answer: We must take control of our lives where we can. In this chapter, we're going to chart those areas where you can change your life. We're going to talk about diet and exercise, cholesterol, fats and fiber, about smoking and alcohol and other substances that affect your heart for better or for worse. We're going to talk about these things because each of them points to lifestyle changes that can make you a healthier person and thus promise you a longer and a fuller life.

---

3 See James W Reed, M.D., et al., *The Black Man's Guide to Good Health* (Perigree, 1994), pp. 41-67; and Ojeda, Linda, Ph.D., *Her Healthy Heart* (op cit.),pp. 64-65.

CHOLESTEROL REVISITED

Here's a little review. Coronary artery disease occurs when the coronary arteries that feed the heart blood are blocked. When your heart doesn't get enough blood, you may experience chest pressure or pain (angina), shortness of breath (often a symptom of congestive heart failure), or sudden death (that is, heart attack, or sudden myocardial infarction). The arteries are clogged by a substance called plaque, made largely of cholesterol, along with fatty deposits and blood cell elements called platelets. When a doctor diagnoses a patient as having arteriosclerosis, it means that cholesterol has built up in the arteries, causing plaque and thus blocking the blood from reaching the heart.

Therefore, the trouble with cholesterol is that as it increases, so does the risk of coronary artery disease. Indeed, coronary artery disease is mostly a cholesterol metabolism problem. When tests show that your cholesterol is high, doctors have reason to suspect that your risk of heart disease is also high.

> *The trouble with cholesterol is that as it increases so does the risk of coronary artery disease.*

Here's the crunch. African Americans are less likely than whites to have their cholesterol checked. We can all think of reasons why this is so. But our purpose here is to explain why such tests are important and what exactly they tell. To do that, we must say a few words about cholesterol itself.

Cholesterol, though it is not the same as fat, is a fatty-like yellow protein that accumulates in the body in two ways. One cause of excess cholesterol is eating too much food that contains it.

Excess cholesterol can also result from inefficient metabolizing of it—that is, the body doesn't use this fuel, thus suffering from its buildup. Often, this condition itself reflects inadequate exercise. A car uses fuel when it goes, not when it sits in the garage. So it is with you and cholesterol.

Understand that cholesterol in itself isn't bad. The body manufactures its own supply because cholesterol is essential to the formation of the cell membrane, and it is also the backbone chemical used to manufacture hormones, especially sex hormones. Cholesterol causes trouble when an excess amount attaches to a chemical (lipoprotein) that carries cholesterol in our bloodstream and together with it attaches to the cell wall of our arteries. What this boils down to is that we need cholesterol, but when we get too much, it hurts us. The trick here, as in most things, is moderation.

We need cholesterol, but when we get too much, it hurts us.

The excess cholesterol that causes problems is also known as low-density lipoproteins (LDLs). But, as you probably know, there's another kind of cholesterol, commonly known as "good cholesterol" and technically known as high-density lipoproteins (HDLs). Whereas the low-density stuff gets attached to the arterial walls, good protein works in an opposite way: It carries cholesterol out of the arteries, transporting it to the liver, where it is excreted in the form of bile. Although the chemistry involving cholesterol can be complicated, the essential facts are simple enough.

There's "bad" cholestrol (L.D.L) and "good" cholestrol (H.D.L.)

- The higher the level of LDL, the greater the chance of coronary artery disease and the greater the chance of heart attack and death.
- According to a study by the National Heart, Lung and Blood Institute, cutting LDL by 25 percent lowers your risk of getting coronary artery disease by 50 percent.
- Doctors recommend that your total cholesterol count be lower than 200 milligrams per deciliter (that's how it is measured in medical terms).
- Doctors recommend that your total cholesterol count be not much lower than 160 mg/dl. When your total cholesterol drops below 150, lung problems, gastrointestinal problems, and perhaps even cancer may result. (For most of us, though, the problem is not low cholesterol.)
- The ratio of your total cholesterol to HDL should be less than 4. The higher over 4 that ratio gets, the more likely it is that cholesterol is plugging up the arteries.

Maybe one reason why African Americans don't want to have their cholesterol tested is that they don't want to hear what we're now going to tell you. If your cholesterol is higher than 200 mg/dl, you must change your life, and that's never easy. The most obvious way you must change it is to avoid saturated fats, which are the principal source of bad cholesterol. The principal sources of saturated fats include meats like steak, ribs, bacon, sausage, and lunch meat. But large doses are also to be

If your cholesterol is higher than 200 mg/dl you must change your life.

found in milk, butter, cheese, cream, and yogurt. And, of course, foods fried in saturated fats, as they tend to be in fast-food restaurants, are also notorious sources of bad cholesterol.

Food high in saturated fat, fast food in general—let's call it what it is: junk *food—offers little nutritional value but much in lethal value.*

So here's Kenya in the midst of her mother's birthday barbecue. How is she to announce these unwelcome truths to her relatives and friends? This food makes people happy, gives them a sense that they're getting something out of life, no matter how tough things may be going in other areas. And one reason that fast-food restaurants are found on the street corners in African American communities is that many people turn to such restaurants for a quick fix, something to feel good about. And, of course, they're easy and convenient.

Though we can understand why people eat badly, we must still insist that they are eating badly—in fact, they're eating in a way that is killing them. Because that's the simple truth. Food high in saturated fat, fast food in general—let's call it what it is: junk food—offers little nutritional value but much in lethal value. It may be convenient, and it may seem to be a way to deal with stress, but it's a suicidal way.

The ironic fact is that, were it not for bad diet and other kinds of neglect or abuse of the body, African Americans ought to have healthier hearts than white Americans. African Americans—both men and women, though men more than women—have been blessed with higher levels of HDL (that is, good cholesterol) than other races. Despite that advantage, risk

The ironic fact is that were it not for bad diet and other kinds of neglect or abuse of the body, African Americans ought to have healthier hearts than white Americans.

factors result in high rates of coronary artery disease among African Americans. These risk factors include hypertension (high blood pressure), smoking, inactivity, obesity, and diet unhealthy for the heart. To us, the special purpose of this book is to restore African Americans to the exceptional good health that our biological makeup promises us.

Let's start with the good stuff—HDL. Exercise increases it, and we'll have more to say about that in a later chapter. Alcohol in moderation increases it: No more than two glasses of red wine per day, or an ounce to an ounce and a half of other alcohol, can be just what the doctor ordered. (Obviously, the alcohol prescription does not apply if you are alcoholic.) While estrogen replacement therapy may possibly help also, studies are still inconclusive. But probably the ideal prescription is weight reduction, which, of course, is one of the fringe benefits of exercise.

You already know what decreases HDL: smoking, obesity, inactivity—and (a new one) steroid use. The increasing use of steroids by athletes and body builders may increase muscle mass, but it carries great risks.

Lowering bad cholesterol, or LDL, is primarily a matter of diet. One simple change that carries great benefit is to cook with monounsaturated fats like canola oil or olive oil, which lower the bad cholesterol and raise the good.

Fish is good for you. In particular, salmon, mackerel, tuna, and sardines are rich with omega-3 fatty acids, which are known to increase HDL.

Soluble fiber also increases HDL, and it's easy to find in apples, carrots, beans, prunes, and bran, whether in the form of breakfast cereals like oatmeal or oat bran muffins.

Finally, antioxidants lower LDL: vitamins A, C, and E are effective antioxidants, but fruits and vegetables (garlic and onions especially), and, as we said, alcohol in moderate quantities, are also good sources.

We've given you a lot of information. Let's try to sum it up. Cholesterol is divided into two types, LDL and HDL. LDL, the bad type of cholesterol, causes coronary arteriosclerosis. To decrease your LDLs, decrease the saturated fats in your diet. That means cutting down on meat, lard, cheese, and butter.

HDL, ordinarily higher in African Americans, is good cholesterol because it helps "cleanse" the body of LDL. We want it to be at the level of 60 mg/dl or above and can usually achieve that level through the right diet, which means monounsaturated oils, fish, fiber, lots of fruit and vegetables, including garlic and onions, and a moderate amount of alcohol. Obviously, if you are alcoholic or have a family history of alcoholism, or if you have suffered liver damage, alcohol should have no place in your diet. Further, for women, more than two drinks of red wine or hard liquor per day can lead to breast cancer and other problems. If you are predisposed to breast cancer because of family history or because you have been treated for it in the past, it's essential that you restrict your alcohol consumption to no more than two ounces a day. Remember that alcohol is just one of the ways to increase HDL.

Limit fried food altogether, or, if you do fry, use olive oil or canola oil. Limit both butter and margarine. Each has its own risks. Load up your diet with fresh fruit and vegetables. Substitute fish for meat as often as you can.

We don't expect absolute virtue in these matters. If you eat right most of the time, you can afford to have a steak on that special occasion. But it isn't necessary to feel that you're eating a prison diet the rest of the time. With only a little extra effort, you can eat tasty and nutritious food without adding to your risk of heart disease.

If you eat right most of the time, you can afford to have a steak on that special occasion.

There are a number of cookbooks that will help you start and maintain heart-healthy diets. Check these out, compare them, and choose the one you like: Wilbert Jones's *The New Soul Food Cookbook* (Birch Lane Press, *1996),* and Danella Carter's *Down-Home Wholesome: 300 Low-Fat Recipes from a New Soul Kitchen* (Penguin, 1998), Jonell Nash's *Low-Fat Soul* (Ballantine Books, 1998).

FATS

The books recommended above emphasize that to keep the fat content low you must watch not only what you cook but what kind of fat you cook it in. Monounsaturated fats, the good fats, are found in olive oil and canola oil. Try them both and see which you and your family prefer. In either case, if your family notices a change in taste the first day, they'll stop noticing it by the second. And remember that even monounsaturated fats need to be used in moderation.

While we're on the subject of fat, you'll recall that we advised you earlier to limit both butter and margarine. Most people know that butter and other cream products are major sources of bad cholesterol, but what's wrong with margarine? Margarine, researchers have discovered recently, is a source of still another kind of fat called trans-fatty acids—a bad fat because it raises total cholesterol and LDL levels at the same time as it lowers the HDL or good cholesterol levels. Trans-fats are found not only in margarine itself but also in cookies, pies, cakes, frostings, chips, and many fast foods. If there were devils in science, trans-fats would be one of them.

You'll also help yourself and your family satisfy fat needs by eating fish, which, you'll recall, contain omega-3 fatty acids. If trans-fats are the devil, omega-3 fatty acids are a kind of guardian angel. They not only decrease LDL but also increase HDL and lower blood pressure. So fish, especially salmon and mackerel (baked or grilled but not fried), is not only an excellent substitute for meat but healthy in itself.

FREE RADICALS

Fats are not the only bad actors in the coronary artery drama. There are also chemicals called free radicals, normally found in our bloodstream, that attach themselves to LDLs by a process called oxygenation. When that happens, free radicals damage the arterial wall of the coronary arteries and thus clog them.

The free radicals can be held in check by elements called antioxidants, which we mentioned above. Probably the best sources of these are fruits and vegetables, especially colorful ones. Among vitamin supplements, vitamins A (beta carotene), C, and E are the most widely used antioxidants. But antioxidants are also available through minerals such as selenium, copper, zinc, and manganese. And, as you know, red wine also contains antioxidants. That is one reason why, despite their love of fat-laden sauces and rich foods, with the help of red wine and fresh fruits and vegetables, the French have healthier hearts than we do.

FIBER

There's truth in the old adage about an apple a day keeping the doctor away.

Fruits and vegetables are not only a source of antioxidants; they also provide us with fiber. Though some recent studies deny this, the consensus for the past forty years or so is that fiber reduces both total cholesterol and LDL, and that, therefore, high-fiber diets are a good way to prevent not only heart disease but also hypertension, diabetes, hemorrhoidal disease, constipation, and colon cancer.

Good sources of fiber include grains, beans, barley, soybeans, fruits, and vegetables. And it turns out that there's truth in the old adage about an apple a day keeping the doctor away. Apples are one of those miracle foods that lowers LDL and increases HDL.

SPECIFIC DIETS

You may wish to put to use the information we've been giving you by following a heart-healthy diet plan. We'll review two of these and say a word about a third. If you are ready for something more extreme than an ordinary, healthy low-fat diet, you may want to consider following Dr. Dean Ornish's program.[4]

---

4 Dr. Ornish has published several books, including *Stress, Diet and Your Health (Holt & Rinehart, 1987), Dr. Dean Ornish's Program for Reversing Heart Disease (Ivy Books, 1996), and Everyday Cooking with Dr. Dean Ornish: 150 Easy, Low-Fat, High-Flavor Dishes* (Harper Collins, 1997).

Dr. Ornish has demonstrated through solid research that patients whose high fat and cholesterol put them at high risk of coronary artery disease can become healthy again by going on extremely low-fat diets, consisting largely of vegetables. He has shown that among people suffering from coronary artery disease, an extremely low-fat diet sharply reduces plaque buildup in the arteries. Keeping your fat intake low lessens the danger that you will suffer from coronary artery disease.

Keeping your fat intake low lessens the danger that you will suffer from coronary artery disease.

Dr. Ornish's diet, low-fat and vegetarian, along with moderate exercise and stress-reducing techniques like meditation, not only can help control coronary artery disease but in some cases may reverse it. But we want to supply a cautious note here. Tough programs like the Dean Ornish diet should be used with caution, and always under a physician's or a registered dietitian's guidance. As we've said before, the point is that we need some fat and cholesterol in our diets. Every cell membrane contains fat and cells don't function unless there's enough of both these substances. Remember that when you lower the overall fat content in your diet, the LDL cholesterol will go down but so will the HDL (the good cholesterol). That's why any extreme low-fat diet should be monitored. Women especially are vulnerable to the side effects of fat deprivation, whose symptoms may include low energy, dry skin, brittle nails, loss of hair, nervousness, confusion, irritability, and menstrual problems. Yes, keep the fat content of your diet low, but with the help of your doctor, monitor it to ensure that it doesn't get too low.

A second well-known low-fat diet is the DASH (Dietary Approaches to Stop Hypertension) diet. The National Heart, Lung and Blood Institute (NHLBI) recommends it to patients with blood pressures in the range of 140 to 150 systolic over 90 to 99 diastolic. Indeed, they often recommend patients with blood pressures in this range try this diet before resorting to medications.

The DASH diet is a bit less extreme and more tolerable than the Ornish diet. It allows 30 percent of total calories to be from fat, as opposed to the 10 percent allowed by the Ornish diet. Further, it permits you to eat red meat, poultry, and fish a few times a week. So does the Mediterranean diet, which, most generous of them all, allows you 40 percent of your total calories in the form of fat. (Any number of books are available for both these diets. For the DASH diet, try, for example, Robert C. Atkins, Dr. Atkins' *New Diet Revolution* (Harper, 1997). For the Mediterannean diet, two popular books are: Nancy Harmon Jenkins, *The Mediterranean Cookbook* (Bantam, Doubleday, Dell, 1994) and Maher A. Abbas, *Olive Oil Cookery: The Mediterranean Diet* (Book Publishing Company, 1995).

The bottom line is that any one of these diets is preferable to the fast food, heavy meat, and saturated fat diet common to African Americans. Low-fat diets, exercise, and stress-relieving exercises—that's the combination through which you can help control and even reverse coronary artery disease.

SUBSTANCES THAT AFFECT THE HEART

Alcohol

We've already spoken about alcohol, but because it's an important subject, we'll talk about it once more. Alcoholism has become a serious problem in the African American community. Rates of alcoholism used to be lower among African Americans than among whites, but this is no longer the case. Not only are African Americans at high risk for alcoholism and alcohol-related disease, but, according to *The Black Man's Guide to Good Health,*[5] drinking problems in African American men usually have a later onset—usually after age thirty—than in white men, for whom heavy and problematic drinking is most evident among younger men. Reed and his colleagues speculate that "this pattern of late onset, if it leads to prolonged heavy consumption, may put us at great risk for chronic diseases related to alcohol consumption"—diseases like congestive heart failure, alcoholic fatty liver, hepatitis, liver cirrhosis, and esophageal cancer. We hardly have to add that alcohol also can lead to devastating problems in the workplace, in relationships, and at home. When Kenya saw the packed liquor stores in Indianapolis, she recognized the potential for wrecked lives.

For women, alcohol presents special problems. Multiple studies have shown that as little as two glasses a day can lead to liver disease and breast cancer. This is true of both black and white women.

Moderate alcohol consumption—5 ounces or less of wine, 12 ounces or less of beer, or 1 1/2 ounces of hard liquor a day—can be beneficial to the heart by increasing HDLs. But if there's a history of alcoholism in your family, or you have liver problems, or you are on medications that don't mix well with alcohol, or you are at risk for breast cancer, 8 to 10 ounces of pure grape juice a day can do the same job. So, too, can plain old aspirin. (But talk to your doctor about aspirin. If you suffer certain medical condi-

5 James. W. Reid, M.D., et al.(Perigree, 1994), p. 235.

tions, he will not recommend them.) Both alcohol and aspirin help inhibit platelets from clogging up coronary arteries.

Tea, whether black or green, is also beneficial to the heart if drunk in moderation. Black and green tea both contain antioxidants that help prevent clogging of the arteries. Black tea has, in addition, heavy amounts of vitamin E. Green tea contains an antioxidant called "catechizes," thought to be as effective as the antioxidants found in wine.

Coffee

Coffee may contribute to heart problems. Although no studies to date conclusively link coffee to heart disease, research does suggest that caffeine, a powerful stimulant, can lead to heart palpitations or a temporary increase in blood pressure, and, further, to panic attacks, anxiety, and insomnia. (Although tea also contains caffeine, the amount per cup is considerably lower than that of a cup of coffee.)

If you are a coffee drinker, remember that you should not drink more than three cups a day. If heart symptoms occur, back off to one cup, or, if your doctor recommends, give up caffeine altogether. It is best to brew by the filter method. Coffee is usually treated with chemicals that may increase cholesterol and fats in your bloodstream. Filtering helps remove these chemicals. In our view, you'll probably feel better—calmer and steadier—if you kick the habit altogether. And if you experience heart palpitations or any of the symptoms listed above, you should stop drinking coffee.

Cocaine

Cocaine is a big problem in the United States today, and an even bigger problem in our African American community. Its victims are black and white, rich and poor, educated and uneducated. In the past several years, cocaine deaths among African Americans have almost tripled. Cocaine tears up families and destroys people. It drains financial resources.

But for us the central issue is that, because cocaine constricts the blood vessels, it can hurt the heart. It can cause dangerous arrhythmias (abnormal heartbeats that often lead to sudden death). A cocaine user isn't likely to do the things that keep the heart healthy, like exercising, eating fruits and vegetables, and maintaining a good diet generally, and keeping his or her life as free of stress as circumstances allow. So the user is inclined toward digestive disorders, emaciation, and impotence. And because cocaine acts on our central nervous system, changes the way we think, and can cause hallucinations, a cocaine user can be unpredictable, capable of violence and brutal crimes.

Nicotine

Smoking would be silly if it weren't so serious. What makes us stick that tube of ground weed into our mouths and inhale? By now, the answer is pretty obvious. Powerful advertising, a powerful narcotic (nicotine), and deliberate concealment of facts got us hooked. Worse yet, as African Americans, we got hooked on the worst that the tobacco industry had to offer—mentholated cigarettes—in which the menthol masks the especially high nicotine and tar content. (About 76% of black cigarette smokers smoke menthol cigarettes, as against 24% of whites.)[6] People smoke metholated cigarettes because that allows them to smoke more and inhale more deeply without experiencing irritation. Don't be fooled. You may not feel it but your body does. The more you smoke, the deeper you inhale, the more

6 *The Black Man's Guide,* p. 32.

likely you are to suffer damage to your lungs and circulatory system that will lead to lung cancer, heart disease, and stroke.

Indeed, smoking is one big reason why the African American community has been so hard hit by coronary disease, hypertension and stroke, as well as by lung and other cancers. Sure, as Kenya noted, cigarette billboards are on all the major corners. Yes, the manufacturers especially want *your* business. But know that cigarettes are one of the leading killers of African American people. Then you will understand what those billboards are saying to you. Here's a diagram that gives you the picture:

How much greater is the risk for smokers of dying from a major disease?

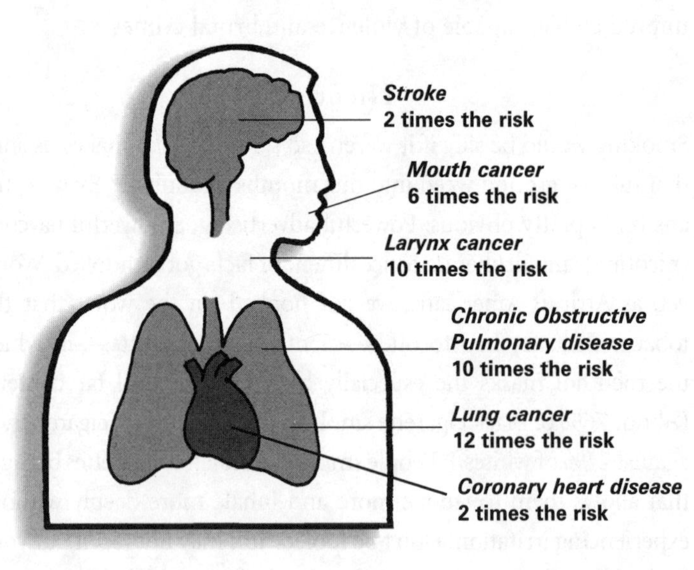

Reprinted with permission from *The Black Man's Guide to Good Health,* by James W. Reed, M.D., F.A.C.P., Neil B. Shulman, M.D., and Charlene Shucker

And here are a few more facts about the effects of nicotine:

- Smokers are twice as likely to suffer strokes (which, incidentally, is another major cause of death among African American men and women).
- Cancer of the mouth is 6 times more likely to happen; of the voice box, 10 times; of the lung, 12 times.
- Lung destruction causing emphysema or obstructive disease is 10 times more likely to happen.
- Smoking not only can cause the blood vessels around the heart to vasoconstrict (get smaller), and therefore be predisposed to close, but it also affects vessels that carry blood to the skin, thereby decreasing nutrients and causing premature wrinkling. (Sure, you've seen it in smokers you know.)
- Smoking increases the risk that vascular disease will lead to gangrene and amputation, especially if the patient also suffers from diabetes.
- Smoking can suppress your immune system, and thus lead to colds and infections.

The picture for women is even worse. A 55-year-old woman who smokes is at greater risk of having heart disease and of suffering a heart attack than a 55-year-old man who smokes. Women who smoke will start menopause earlier and, as a result, the protective effect that estrogen provides against heart disease is lost. In addition, in women more than men, HDL is decreased as a result of smoking. And, finally, smoking increases bad cholesterol (LDL), so the chance of coronary artery disease is increased.

If you want a worst-case scenario from the perspective of a cardiologist or cardiac surgeon, it's this: an obese, diabetic woman who smokes. She is least likely to recover without complications from a heart attack or from bypass surgery.

For men and women, smoking is the worst thing you can do to your heart and to your body generally. Smokers have a 70 percent chance of suffering from heart disease, heart attack, or stroke; if you have coronary artery disease and smoke, your chance of sudden death is two to four times higher than if you don't. Smokers who have a coronary bypass operation and continue to smoke afterward are more likely to require a second bypass surgery, a more dangerous operation than the first. That's because smoking is one of the quickest and most reliable ways of reblocking the newly created bypass graft.

Smokers have a 70% chance of suffering heart disease, heart attack, or stroke; if you have coronary artery disease and smoke, your chance of sudden death is 2-4 times higher than if you don't.

In case you're not getting our drift, smoking is the worst abuse you can inflict on your body in general and on your heart specifically. What makes that fact painful is, of all the problems we've addressed, cigarette smoking is within your direct ability to control. You can't, by your own efforts, stop having hypertension (though you can certainly improve it), and you can't, by your own efforts, stop having diabetes (though you can certainly improve it). But you can stop smoking.

Even if you've smoked all your grown life, stopping will make you healthier. We don't pretend if you've smoked for years and then stop that your lungs and heart will be as good as new. They won't. But stopping will improve them immediately and significantly. A smoker who has given the habit up for a year is fifty percent less likely to suffer coronary artery disease or a heart attack than one who continues to smoke. After abstaining for five years or more, a former smoker's chance of dying of lung cancer is sixty percent lower than that of a current smoker. And after fifteen years, his chance of getting lung cancer is no higher than a nonsmoker's. A woman who has quit smoking for as little as two years, should she suffer coronary artery disease, has the same chance of strong recovery as a nonsmoker.

Stopping smoking will improve your heart and lungs in ways so immediate and so significant—and improve your chances of long life so dramatically—that you'd be a fool not to stop.

Now add the secondary advantages of stopping. Of course, you'll smell better. If you're male, your sexual performance will improve. You'll cough less and get fewer pulmonary infections. And, if you are say, a two-to-three-pack-a-day smoker, each year $1,000 to $1,500 will stay in your pocket.

One last fact: If you're around smokers, even if you yourself are not a smoker, you will be injured by smoke exhaled by those near you who are smoking. There's simply no escaping it: If there's a smoker in the house, everyone in that house is at risk.

Yes, smoking is an addiction, like cocaine or alcohol. You depend on it psychologically and physically. You will suffer withdrawal symptoms if you try to quit. You may want some outside help in dealing with them. Although plenty of people have quit on their own, you have the highest chance of kicking nicotine if you turn to others for support. Maybe it's simply that, by making your intention public by telling someone else about it, you strengthen your resolve.

The most obvious place to turn is to your doctor. He or she can help you both by counseling and by prescribing medications like nicotine patches. Your doctor can also put you in touch with local support groups. If you don't have a doctor, there are other people you can turn to. Smokers Anonymous (P.O. Box 25335, West Los Angeles, CA 90025) provides information to people who wish to quit smoking and can get you in touch with a local group. The American Cancer Society publishes a free handbook called *The Quit Book,* which you can get by writing to them at 4 West 35th Street, New York, NY 10001. And the American Lung Association sponsors a handbook called *Freedom from Smoking for You and Your Family,* which you can order by writing to them at 1740 Broadway, New York, NY 10019.

Although there's help available and we recommend that you take advantage of it, in the end, it's your habit and you're the one who must break it.

Remember that although some of these symptoms are tough to beat, there's a simple truth that gives you an advantage: However fiercely a symptom hits you, if you hold out for 5 minutes, it will pass. Just 5 minutes! You can do that standing on your head.

Here are few more suggestions for kicking your habit:

1. Set a date and time for quitting and stick to it.
2. Picture yourself as a person who has successfully stopped smoking.

3. Chew gum, eat plenty of fruits and vegetables, and absolutely avoid coffee and alcohol. You know how comfortably cigarettes go with coffee and alcohol.
4. Don't let your body dwell on cigarettes. Keep your hands busy. And give your body another focus: Play sports, exercise, or take frequent cold showers or baths.
5. While you're working on this big change, buy some new clothes, get your teeth cleaned, maybe even change your hairstyle. The fact is, you've chosen to start your life over, and like a good actor, you need a few props or costume changes to help you with this new character.
6. Read all you can about the effects of smoking and about people who have quit. Maybe find a friend who also wants to quit. You can help each other out. And avoid friends who do smoke, or politely ask them not to smoke around you. If they're truly your friends, they'll be glad to oblige.
7. If you are religious and believe in the Lord, ask your minister and fellow church members to pray for you and ask the Lord for help in this endeavor.
8. Reward yourself each day that you don't smoke. Not with fattening food, please. You already know about that. But give yourself a treat that's good for your body or your soul. You might give yourself a bigger reward for each week or month that you've kept yourself clean of nicotine.
9. When possible, avoid the smoking sections of restaurants and airports.
10. Keep notes in your pocket or in a little laminated card stating that you've quit and the reasons why.

11. Listening to music, reading a book, and working at a hobby are all ways of resisting the urge to smoke.
12. Keep telling yourself you can quit. You can. You will.

So there it is: the sermon Kenya might have preached to her friends and family on the night of her mother's birthday celebration. It asks big changes of us—in the way we eat and cook, in the things we put into our bodies. What it promises is that, by making these changes, we can become the healthy, vigorous and courageous people that God meant us to be.

Chapter 13

CHOOSING WHAT TO EAT

SOUL FOOD IS LOADED with salt and fat, but it's a deeply rooted part of our heritage. Where do we go from here? Let's go first to history. As slaves, our African forebears were given scraps of meat, scant rations of staples, and the produce they were able to grow for themselves. They transformed those bare bones into hearty meals full of flavor and made with love. Such meals were among the few joys our ancestors were allowed to relish. And, because they did back-breaking work in the fields, high-fat, high-calorie meals were the proper nourishment. They had no trouble burning off the fat.

We still love the meals passed down from our ancestors. But today we know that for our hearts' sakes we must cut down not only on calorie intake but on our consumption of saturated fats, cholesterol, and sodium as well. We must also increase our intake of fruits and vegetables, whole grains, and, in the place of butter and lard, monounsaturated fats. In this chapter we're going to talk to you about a sensible way to do this.

We don't pretend that it's easy to change your eating habits. And of course we can't make that change happen. Only you can do that. But maybe we can make it a little easier by not spending too much time talking about what you shouldn't eat. Instead, we'll lead you toward a way of having your cake and eating it too. We want you to eat what tickles your palate and to still stay healthy, to chuck out the fat without chucking out the flavor.

Only you can change your eating habits.

THE FOOD GUIDE PYRAMID

We've spoken favorably about several diets, including DASH (Dietary Approaches to Stop Hypertension). The trouble is that sticking to a diet is a little like forcing yourself to be good. You know that your real virtues aren't the result of forcing yourself. In the case of behavior, just as forced goodness is likely to erupt eventually into some kind of nastiness, so diets seem to invite binges and to plunge the dieter into an endless cycle of being "good" and then being "bad."

We don't think that diets work for most people, and we know that some diets are worse than others. Some red flags to watch out for are as follows:

- Any diet that restricts or eliminates a food group
- Any diet that has you eating the same foods or the same meals repeatedly (for example, the grapefruit diet)

- Any diet that claims you can lose more than 1 to 2 pounds per week

Eating healthy is not about that, nor is it about spending a fortune buying special foods or special shakes or special pills. Eating healthy allows you to eat all foods, and even allows you to splurge a little at a party or over the holidays. Eating healthy allows you to eat all the things you like—but in moderation.

The closest that this book will come to prescribing a "diet" will be to recommend that you be guided by the food pyramid below.

That little chart clears up a lot of confusion about nutrition. Follow it and you'll meet your nutritional needs while painlessly reducing your intake of fats and sodium. The pyramid suggests but doesn't prescribe what to eat each day. And, as we'll show you, even soul food, with some modification, fits into the pyramid.

The pyramid lays out the five food groups we all positively need, and the one (fats, oils, and sweets) that we need to be wary of. Each of the five groups provides some of the nutrients you need, but none of the groups provide all. And no single group can take the place of another. For good health, we need them all.

The pyramid also indicates the number of servings recommended for each group—those we can eat most abundantly at the bottom, and those we need to eat more sparingly toward the top. As to how many servings of anything you need, that depends on your age, sex, and size and on how active you are. Servings are a rough way of calculating the more fundamental measure—the calorie. The calorie is a measure of heat, which you can also think of as a measure of fuel, or food energy. When we take in more calories than we can burn, they turn to fat.

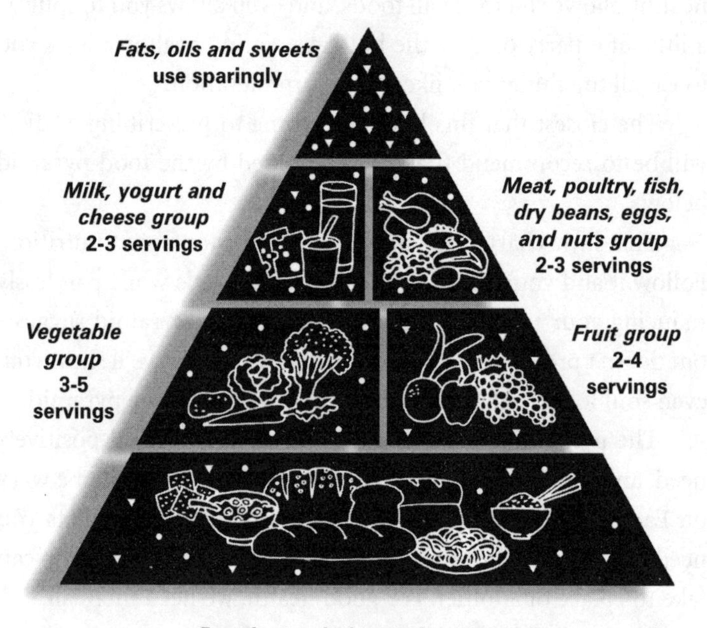
The Food Pyramid:
A guide to daily food choices
Fats, oils and sweets
use sparingly
Milk, yogurt and
cheese group
2-3 servings
Meat, poultry, fish,
dry beans, eggs,
and nuts group
2-3 servings
Vegetable
group
3-5
servings
Fruit group
2-4
servings
Bread, cereal, rice, and pasta group
6-11 servings
Fat, naturally occurring and added
Sugars, added

Here is a rough estimate of what we need:

- 1,600 calories for most women and older adults
- 2,200 calories for kids, teen age girls, active women, and most men
- 2,800 calories for teenage boys and active men

If you're in one of the groups with lower needs, select from the pyramid the lower number of servings. Simply match the number of servings with your place in the above three categories. Concerning the actual amount for meat, it will range from 5 to 7 ounces, depending on your group.

Pregnant and nursing women, along with teens and young adults up to age 24, should drink three servings of milk daily. And, of course, there are other special cases. But for our general purposes, a serving is indicated in the chart below. If you eat a larger portion, it is more than one serving. Thus, while a slice of bread is one serving, a hamburger bun is two. For mixed foods, simply estimate the food group servings of the main ingredients. Thus, a large piece of sausage pizza would count in the bread group (crust), the milk group (cheese), the meat group (sausage), and the vegetable group (tomato sauce). (But, if you're determined to eat right, you could order one with broccoli, mushrooms, etc., and get the benefit of some vegetables. A helping of beef stew would count in the meat group and the vegetable group.)

What counts as a serving? Here it is:

WHAT COUNTS AS A SERVING

Bread, Cereal, Rice, and Pasta Group

1 slice of bread
1 tortilla
1/2 cup cooked rice, pasta, or cereal
1 ounce ready-to-eat cereal
1/2 hamburger roll, bagel, or English muffin
3–4 crackers (small)
1 pancake (4 inch)
1/2 croissant (large)
1/2 doughnut or Danish (medium)
1/16 cake (average):
2 cookies (medium)
1/12 pie (2 crusts, 8")

Vegetable Group

1/2 cup raw or cooked vegetables
1 cup raw, leafy vegetable
3/4 cup vegetable juice
1/2 cup scalloped potatoes
1/2 cup potato salad
10 french fries

Fruit Group

1 piece fruit or melon wedge

Milk, Yogurt, and Cheese Group

1 cup milk or yogurt
1 1/2 ounces natural cheese

continued on the next page

What counts as a serving, continued

Fruit Group	Milk, Yogurt, and Cheese Group
3/4 cup fruit juice	2 ounces processed cheese
1/2 cup chopped, cooked, or canned fruit	1 1/2 cup ice cream or ice milk
1/4 cup dried fruit	1/4 cup dried fruit
1 cup frozen yogurt	

Meat, Poultry, Fish, Dry Beans,	Eggs,Fats, Oils, Sweets, and Nuts Group
2 1/2 to 3 ounces cooked lean beef, pork lamb, veal, poultry, or fish	Use sparingly
1/2 cup cooked beans or 1 egg or 2 tablespoons peanut butter or 1/3 cup nuts all count as 1 ounce of meat. (3 ounces of meat is about the size of a deck of cards, or the size of your palm)	
Lean beef choices: round tip, top round, eye of round, top loin, tenderloin, sirloin	

FATS

We talked in the last chapter about fats, but because they're so important we'll talk about them again. As you know, there are two types of fat: saturated and unsaturated. The saturated fats are most likely to result in cholesterol and plaque in your arteries. To make things just a bit more confusing, unsaturated fats are divided into two categories: polyunsaturated and monounsaturated. The monounsaturated fats are the good guys.

Although most foods contain several types of fat, we can classify food according to their predominant kind. Thus, saturated fats are found in animal products such as meat, whole milks, and lard, and in dairy products like cheese, ice cream, and butter. Certain vegetable oils, like palm, palm kernel, coconut oils, and cocoa butter, are sources of saturated fats. This latter group is sometimes referred to as tropical fats. Tropical fats, though heavily saturated, don't contain cholesterol. But, like all saturated fats, they raise blood cholesterol.

That's what saturated fats do: While they may not themselves contain cholesterol, they raise the cholesterol in the blood. A food like potato chips can be "cholesterol-free" but still very high in saturated fats. Keep in mind that the now common marketing ploy that a food is cholesterol-free may simply mean that you need to take a closer look at the nutritional label.

Despite the danger that fats can pose to the body, the body needs fat. It is a good energy source, it promotes a healthy nervous system, and it protects against mental decline. That need is best satisfied with monounsaturated fats. Instead of raising your bad cholesterol level, they actually lower it. In addition, they increase your good cholesterol.

Olive oil is an excellent source, as are peanut oil and canola oil. That's why we recommend that you use them as much as possible in your cooking rather than saturated fats. Monounsaturated fats are often found in many fish and seafood (we've mentioned mackerel and salmon as an especially good source), in nuts, olives, and avocados.

Polyunsaturated fats are found in safflower, sunflower, corn, soybean, cottonseed, and sesame seeds. They are too effective as cholesterol busters. They lower bad cholesterol, but they also lower good cholesterol.

If you want a physical image to guide you, think of it this way. The more solid a fat is at room temperature, the more saturated it is. Lard and shortening are very solid and therefore very saturated. Stick margarine and butter are still pretty solid and are very saturated. Tub margarine and butters are better, oils are better still, and cooking sprays are best.

Now consider omega-3 fatty acids. These are found in fish and fish oils and in canola. Canola is so effective in lowering blood cholesterol as well as triglyceride levels that we recommend it even above olive oil. (Omega-3 fatty acids are also found in soybeans, certain nuts and seeds.)

Omega three fatty acids are found in fish, fish oils and canola.

You can buy fish oils in health food stores, but a better and cheaper source is a frequent diet of fish and shellfish (at least once or twice a week). Remember that even the fattiest fish—salmon—is far leaner than the leanest beef. That's true also of shrimp, scallops, lobster, etc. Some people avoid them because of their cholesterol content. But the good they'll do with their fatty acids far outweighs the cholesterol. (Just go easy on the butter and tartar sauce.)

If you put your reading glasses on and go down the list of ingredients in processed or snack food you have in the cupboard, you'll run into another oil, usually called partially hydrogenated vegetable oil. Now that you know it, limit your use of it. Though it begins as a safe vegetable oil, it is hydrogenated so that the product can sit long on the shelf, and the hydrogenation process makes it become very saturated. These fats, also known as trans-fatty acids, not only cause cholesterol to increase but they may pose a risk for certain types of cancers.

Eating the right kind of fat can lower your risks of coronary artery disease and heart attack. But fat is fat, and it means calories. If we eat more calories than we burn off, the extra calories are stored as body fat, no matter where those calories come from. People know this, presumably, and that's why we've seen so many fat-free products in the grocery markets. Unfortunately, they don't seem to do much good. While they've helped Americans cut their fat intake from 36 percent to 34 percent of their average daily calories, during the same period we've gained 8 pounds per person!

The problems may be that fat-free foods, whether as meals or snacks, don't fill us as fatty foods do. So we end up eating more of them, and, in the process, we take in more calories. Don't fall into the illusion that because a food is fat-free you can eat all you want. That could be a heavy mistake.

Another recent fad has been fat substitutes that deliver some of the desirable qualities of fat but add fewer calories. Some of them—cellulose gel Apical, guar gum, and gum Arabic—have been around for a long time and are considered safe. But there are also new synthetic fat substitutes on the market, and we know little about their long-term effects.

Probably the best known of these is Olestra. It passes from the body without leaving behind any calories from fat. (Keep in mind that foods containing these products still contain calories that come from protein and carbohydrates.) For some people, it doesn't pass through the body without leaving behind cramps and mild to severe diarrhea. It also depletes the body of vitamins A, K, D, and E, though the FDA (Food and Drug Administration) now requires that the missing vitamins be added back to foods containing Olestra products. Nevertheless, there seems reason to practice caution about food containing Olestra.

There are a number of other such fat substitutes, but some of them are still high in saturated fats and some are high in calories. On the whole, we recommend that you use these substitutes sparingly and with some caution

SODIUM

Time for everything you always wanted to know about salt. The main thing you know already: If you have high blood pressure or if you're salt-sensitive, you need to follow a low-salt diet—2,000 to 3,000 milligrams a day—because salt can make hypertension worse. For the rest of us, a "no added salt" diet works fine. It allows from 3,000 to 4,000 milligrams a day, which is a liberal allowance.

> *If you have high blood pressure or if you're salt-sensitive, you need to follow a low salt diet.*

While most of us haven't given much thought to whether we are salt-sensitive, African Americans tend to be so more than whites. So, playing the odds, and given the very high rate of hypertension among African Americans, you're probably doing yourself a favor to cut back on salt, if you don't cut it out altogether.

That's actually easier to do than you might think. The taste for salt is learned, which means that it can be unlearned. Within two months of not adding salt to your food, your taste buds will have become so sensitized that salted foods will taste oversalted. At that point, you'll find that your tongue is taking in all kinds of new taste pleasures that previously were masked by salt.

Many prepared foods contain high levels of sodium.

The hard part about reducing salt is that many prepared foods contain sodium, although you may not think of them as especially salty. A half cup of chocolate-flavored instant pudding, for example, has 470 milligrams of sodium, and two slices of bacon have 245 milligrams. Cheese, cured meats, canned soups, commercial tomato sauce, many snack and fast foods, foods that contain monosodium glutamate (common in Chinese food), and baked foods with baking soda and baking powder are all high in sodium.

We recommend that you make your own dishes. That way, you are within your power to feed yourself and your family what's good for all of you and to control the salt. If, after a while on a no-salt-added diet, you still have a craving, you can afford the occasional luxury of salted nuts or chips. But you may find that you don't need salt at all. Using herbs and spices will give your food a new kind of zest that you and your family may in the end find tastier than salt.

Using herbs and spices will give your food a new kind of zest.

FIBER

Another nutritional gift you can give your heart is fiber. (To call fiber "nutritional" is a little misleading, because not all fiber is digested. Unsoluble fiber passes through the intestines, drawing water with it, and is eliminated.) High-fiber diets lower cholesterol. One study shows that among two groups of people on a reduced-fat diet, those who took 25 grams of fiber a day lowered their cholesterol by 13 percent; those who didn't, lowered their cholesterol by 9 percent. It isn't known why fiber lowers cholesterol. One theory suggests that it may bind to cholesterol and bile acids in the intestines and prevent the body from absorbing them, so they are excreted with other body wastes.

Fiber helps prevent colon cancer and other intestinal problems.

Because fiber seems to work that way, and because, in addition, it helps prevent colon cancer and other intestinal problems (pectin, a kind of fiber found in apples, grapefruits, and oranges, may specifically protect against heart disease), it's important that you take in 20 to 35 grams daily. Soluble fiber is found in oat bran, beans and other legumes, barley, prunes, and various fruits and vegetables. If you don't keep up your diet with such foods, as recommended by the chart on page 220, you can get fiber in the form of psyllium, a natural grain grown in India and found commercially as Metamucil, Fiberall, and Perdiem.

Because fiber draws water from the body, it's important that you increase your water intake as you increase your fiber intake. It's also true that diets high in fiber can cause bloating and gas. Usually, that problem vanishes once you've made fiber a regular part of your diet. But if you are having trouble with gas, this can be relieved by an enzyme marketed as Beano, which is sold over the counter. If beans—one good source of fiber—are the cause of the problem, add 1/8 teaspoon of baking soda to the water in which you soak the beans.

FIBER CONTENT OF FOODS[1]

Foods	Portion	Fiber (grams)
peas, green	1/2 cup	5.2
kidney beans	1/2 cup	4.5
apple, with skin	1 small	3.9
apricots, with skin	2 medium	1.5
bread, whole wheat	1 slice	2.7
broccoli	1/2 cup	2.4
brown rice, cooked	1 cup	2.4
white rice, cooked	1 cup	2.4
lima beans	1/2 cup	1.4
lettuce	1/2 cup	0.5

1 This table is exerpted from *The Eating Well, Living Well Series* by the staff of the Sarah W. Stedman Center for Nutritional Studies, 1996, by arrangement with Viking Penguin.

VITAMINS AND MINERALS

We treated this subject in a different context when we talked about managing stress. Here we only want to emphasize again that vitamins, whether you get them as part of a good and varied diet, or as supplements purchased at the drug store, are important to the health of your heart. They may also help in preventing or relieving stress. Your doctor can tell you whether he thinks you would be helped by taking vitamin supplements.

NUTRITION AND THE GROCERY STORE

Now that we've established some general principles of nutrition, let's go shopping. The produce is simple. You'll want to pick up lots of fruits, vegetables, whole grains, and low-fat, low-cholesterol dairy products.

Now comes the hard part: How do you know what you're getting when you buy packaged and prepared foods? Uncle Sam's made it easier for you, by requiring that manufacturers tell you what's in a product. The trouble is that they tell you in small print and long lists. But there's no way around it. Either you read the lists, until you've familiarized yourself with the products, or you must rely on advertising claims, which are often false. On the other hand, certain claims can now be made only if the food meets government specifications.

Now we get down to the fine print. Here are some important things to know about the list of ingredients that appears on all packaged food.

- The most helpful parts of the label are the *ingredient list* and the *nutrition facts.*

WHAT THE LABELS MEAN

Label Claim	Definition
Calorie-free	Less than 5 calories
Low calorie	40 calories or less
Light or lite	1/3 fewer calories or 50 percent less fat than the standard product. If more than half the calories are fat, the fat content must be reduced by 50 percent or more.
Light in sodium	50 percent less sodium than the standard product
Fat-free	Less than 1/2 gram fat
Low fat	3 grams or less fat
Cholesterol-free	Less than 2 milligrams cholesterol and 2 grams or less saturated fat
Low cholesterol	20 milligrams or less cholesterol and 2 grams or less saturated fat
Sodium-free	Less than 5 milligrams sodium
Very low sodium	35 milligrams sodium
Low sodium	140 milligrams or less sodium
High fiber	5 grams or more fiber

- Ingredients are listed in order of the amount used, from the most to the least.
- The types of fat—saturated, monounsaturated, or polyunsaturated—and their order on the list are important. Check them. Manufacturers often use two or more types of fat and list them separately farther down the list than they would be if they were grouped together. In that case, fat may not appear to be a major ingredient when it is. Check this.
- Claims that a product contains no cholesterol are misleading. A product free of cholesterol may be very high in fat—even saturated fat! Check this on the list.
- Some products, acceptable in small portions, contribute too much fat to the diet if eaten in large quantities. Check the portion size on the nutritional label.

Before leaving home, make a shopping list that includes enough of the basic and staple food to last until your next planned trip to the store.

Done shopping? We know it took a little longer because you had to read all those labels. But next time it will go faster. Anyway, now you're home and it's time to start thinking about cooking and eating.

Because you're now into low-fat cooking, you will have to make some adjustments. Fat serves several functions: It adds moisture, it carries or enhances flavor, it gives food a certain feel in your mouth, and it makes you feel full. As you make the transition to low-fat cooking, an adjustment you'll need to make so that you and your family won't feel taste deprived is to spark your cooking with new herbs and spices.

Food label guide

Nutrition Facts
Serving Size 1 cup (228g)
Servings Per Container 2

Amount Per Serving
Calories 90 Calories from Fat 30

	% Daily Value*
Total Fat 3g	**5%**
Saturated Fat 0g	**0%**
Cholesterol 0mg	**0%**
Sodium 300mg	**13%**
Total Carbohydrate 13g	**4%**
Dietary Fiber 3g	**12%**
Sugars 3g	
Protein 3g	

Vitamin A 80% • Vitamin C 60%
Calcium 4% • Iron 4%

* Percent Daily Values are based on a 2,000 calorie diet. Your daily values may be higher or lower depending on your calorie needs:

	Calories:	2,000	2,500
Total Fat	Less than	65g	80g
Sat Fat	Less than	20g	25g
Cholesterol	Less than	300mg	300mg
Sodium	Less than	2,400mg	2,400mg
Total Carbohydrate		300g	375g
Dietary Fiber		25g	30g

Calories per gram:
Fat 9 • Carbohydrate 4 • Protein 4

% Daily Value shows how a food fits into a 2,000 calorie reference diet.

Similar food products now have similar serving sizes to make comparisons easier. Serving sizes are based on amounts of food people actually eat.

Daily Values are set by the government and based on current nutrition recommendations. Some labels list the daily values for a daily diet of 2,000 and 2,500 calories. Your own nutrient needs may be less or more.

Nutrient list covers those that are most important to your health.

Only two vitamins, A and C, and two minerals, calcium and iron, are required on food labels. Some food companies voluntarily list other vitamins and minerals found in their food.

Some labels tell the approximate number of calories in a gram of fat, carbohydrate and protein.

Note: Numbers on nutrition labels may be rounded.

Many of these are said to be good for you. But they also taste terrific. Try them out, to see which of them, and which combinations, best please your palate. Just to give you an idea of the range, there's freshly grated ginger, garlic, citrus zest, dry mustard, hot peppers, dried fruits, and dried vegetables like tomatoes that will color and intensify your cooking in ways you never imagined. You'll also find a number of salt-free blends on the spice shelves.

As for the recipes themselves, there's no need to abandon the old ones, although you'll probably want to add some new ones to mark your new cooking style. Most recipes can easily be adapted to lower-fat versions simply by substituting ingredients that are high in total fat, saturated fat, or cholesterol with lower-fat alternatives. Sometimes an ingredient will have to be eliminated altogether because no low-fat alternative is available, or you can just reduce the amount of that high-fat ingredient. We'll show you some cooking methods that make the reduction of fat easier.

Just remember that, while you're learning this new style, you will need to examine each ingredient carefully so that, at each step of your recipe, you can cut the fat. It may be as easy as frying in a nonstick skillet with a spritz of vegetable spray instead of adding globs of butter or oils. Or you may wish to substitute ground turkey for ground beef. The turkey has 50 percent less saturated fat than other ground meats!

Here is a list of substitutions you can make when you're cooking—and some that work even when you're eating out.

LIST OF SUBSTITUTIONS

Instead of	Use
1 tbsp. butter	1 tsp. margarine or 1/4 tbsp. canola, peanut, or olive oil
1 cup butter	3/4 cup canola or olive oil
1 cup shortening	2/3 cup canola or olive oil
1 whole egg	2 egg whites or 1/4 egg substitute
1 cup sour cream	1 cup low-fat yogurt (plain) whole milk skim or 1 percent milk
1 cup cream	evaporated skim milk or evaporated milk
whipped cream or topping containing saturated fat	pressurized whipped cream (2 tbsp.= 1 gram fat, 16 calories)
mayonnaise	lite mayonnaise
ice cream	low-fat frozen yogurt, ice milk, sorbet, ices, etc.
1 oz. baking chocolate	3 tbsp. baking cocoa plus 1 tbsp. oil
cottage cheese	low-fat cottage cheese (but be aware that "low fat" cottage cheese still contains 4% milkfat)
bacon, sausage, hot dogs	Canadian bacon or lean ham

continued on the next page

List of Substitutions, continued

Instead of	**Use**
beef	lean ground round, ground sirloin, turkey, or chicken (10 percent fat)
cheese	low-fat cheese (2 to 6 grams fat/oz).
salad dressing	low-calorie salad dressing
1 can cream soup	homemade white sauce: 1 cup skim milk, 1 tbsp. margarine, 2 tbsp. flour
canned spaghetti sauce	6 oz. tomato paste and 18 oz. water to 1 jar of sauce
potato chips on casseroles	bread crumbs or cereal crumbs (for example, corn flakes)
cakes, cookies, brownies	vanilla wafers, gingersnaps, crackers, fortune cookies, angel food cake, fruit
sausage/pepperoni pizza	vegetarian pizza
packaged lunch meats	thinly sliced deli meats—chicken, beef
croissants	bagels, English muffins, soft pretzels
french fries	homemade oven fries (no more than 1 tsp. oil/serving)
chips	popcorn, pretzels
2-crust pies	one-crust or graham cracker crust

ADDITIONAL COOKING AND DINING TIPS

- Use a minimum amount of fat in cooking.
- Avoid frying and deep-fat frying. Use low-fat cooking methods—bake, broil, microwave, steam, poach, grill.
- Trim fat from meat before and after cooking.
- Remove poultry skin.
- Tenderize lean cuts of meat with marinades, mechanical pounding, or a tenderizer.
- Cook longer at low heat rather than shorter at high heat.
- Use moist heat, adding liquid or using meat's own juices, where appropriate.
- Remove fat from soups and stews by making them a day early, then refrigerating and skimming solid fat.
- Drain all fat from cooked ground beef. Pat with paper towels and wipe out the pan before adding spices, vegetables, etc.
- Make pasta, legumes, rice, or vegetables the focus of the meal instead of meat.
- Use smaller portions of meat, fish, and poultry.
- Include meatless meals using beans and legumes.
- Use nonstick pans or sprays.
- Invest in a sharp knife to remove fat from meat and poultry and to cut thin slices for stir-fry dishes.
- Use nonfat dry milk and skim milk in cooking soups, puddings, casseroles, and muffins.
- Use cheese as a garnish. Sprinkle small amounts on top of casseroles, etc.
- Use herbs, spices, and butter alternatives to flavor vegetables, soups, etc.

We mentioned the excellent book *Low-Fat Soul* in chapter 12, but we want to list here our favorite guides to preparing healthier versions of the foods we love.

- *Ruby's Low-Fat Soul Food Cookbook,* by Ruby Banks.
- *The New Soul Food Cookbook—Healthier Recipes for Traditional Favorites,* by Wilbert Jones (Birch Lane Press, *1996).*
- *Down-Home Wholesome,* by Danella Carter (Penguin, 1998). Ms. Carter's 300 low-fat soul recipes are especially good at replacing or eliminating high-fat flavor bases with heart-friendly alternatives.
- *Low-Fat Soul,* by Jonell Nash (Ballantine Books, 1998). Ms. Nash, the food editor at *Essence* magazine, has put together—in her words—"more than 100 delicious recipes that still have the flava without the fat."

Although you have all this new and interesting work to do in the kitchen, you may want to take a break once in a while and let somebody else do the cooking. But don't let eating out be a reason for abandoning your program of healthy eating. Here are some guidelines:

- Study the menu to identify the healthier items offered.
- Ask for salad dressing on the side. Inquire about fat-free dressings, reduced-calorie dressings, or use lemon juice.
- Request baked or broiled seafood with no butter or ask for margarine on the side and limit the amount you use.
- Order vegetables served without added fat. If you want margarine on your potatoes, use it sparingly.

- Order sandwiches without dressing, bacon, or cheese. (Even fast-food sandwiches can usually be special ordered this way.) Ask for lettuce and tomato to make the sandwich moist.
- Watch portion sizes, particularly with the entree. Many restaurants serve much more than what is needed or healthy.

You get the message, but let us repeat it. You can control what goes into your mouth. Sure, it takes careful planning, shopping, and cooking to establish a low-fat lifestyle. But that should be easy when you keep in mind that it is a lifestyle. Eating is one of life's great pleasures. We don't think that you have to sacrifice that pleasure in order to treat your body with the loving attention it needs. You'll get benefits you never enjoyed when you were eating the bad old way. For one, you'll like the way you look. And, as if that weren't good enough, you'll like the way you feel. What it's all about, after all, is keeping the beat, and if that means eating leaner, it seems a small price to pay.

You can control what you eat.

Afterword

"To take our wellness in hand," in Maya Angelou's words, is a giant step forward in the continuing effort to empower our African American community. To be healthy and strong enables us to express the pride and hope that makes life worth living; it enables us to live longer, more fruitful lives and to share those lives with our families, our churches, and our communities. Good health allows us to partake of life more fully, its wonders and challenges, its struggles and rewards.

This book was written to help you understand heart disease and its treatments. We hope it's done that. We also hope this book will help you take control of your health and understand how to work with the health care system to your own benefit. Knowledge is power. The more knowledge, the greater the power. The longer you live and the more experiences you have, the more you know and the greater your power to help yourself, your family, and your community. Your life matters. Choose to live!

Appendix I

YOUR RIGHTS AS A PATIENT

YOU DON'T LOSE YOUR human rights when you are admitted to a hospital. The best way to defend these rights is to go in with a clear knowledge of the proper treatment and courtesy you are entitled to. Never be afraid to ask questions. Be pleasant but firm, determined but cooperative. The rights to which you are entitled include:

- Your right to know the identity of every doctor, nurse, student, or resident who provides care for you or who contacts you while you are a patient in the hospital.
- Your right to receive complete information about your condition and treatment, and to receive such information confidentially and respectfully.

- Your right to receive all information prior to submitting to any treatment and prior to signing an informed consent agreement.
- Your right to refuse consent.
- Your right to review all records and communication about your treatment.
- Your right to prepare advance directives such as a living will, health care proxy, or power of attorney and for such wishes to be adhered to by the hospital.
- Your right to be informed if the hospital is involved with any type of human experimentation that might affect your care.
- Your right to receive considerate and respectful care.

Appendix 2

LOW FAT SOUL FOOD RECIPES

The following Low Fat Soul Food Recipes are from *The New Soul Food Cookbook* by Wilbert Jones, reprinted by permission of the author and from *Down-Home Wholesome* by Danella Carter, reprinted by permission of Penguin Putnam, Inc.

SOUPS AND SALADS

Black Bean Soup

8 cups

1/2 cup diced celery
1/2 cup diced onion
2 tablespoons crushed fresh garlic
nonstick cooking spray
3 cups dried black beans (rinsed and sorted)
1 teaspoon celery salt
1 teaspoon chili powder
1/2 teaspoon ground red pepper
1/2 cup dry white wine
2 teaspoons Tabasco sauce

1. Over medium-low heat, saute the celery, onion, and garlic for about 10 minutes (or until the vegetables become translucent) in a nonstick skillet sprayed with nonstick cooking spray. Pour the beans, celery salt, chili powder, red pepper, wine, and Tabasco sauce in a large pot.
2. Add the sauteed celery, onions, and garlic to the pot along with 12 cups of water. Over high heat, heat to boiling. Cover the pot, reduce heat to low, and cook for about 3 hours.

Per Serving
Calories: 110
Protein: 6 grams
Carbohydrates: 18 grams
Fat: 1 gram
Sodium: 19 milligrams

Tomato Soup

Makes 6 cups

5 cups fresh tomatoes, skinned and seeded
1/2 cup chopped celery
1/2 chopped onion
1/3 cup skim milk
1 tablespoon brown sugar
1 teaspoon chopped chives
1/2 cup water

1. Blend the tomatoes in a blender for about 2 minutes. Then combine the tomatoes with the celery, onion, milk, sugar, chives, and water in a pot and cook for 10 minutes or until it simmers.

Per Serving
Calories: 40
Protein: 1 gram
Carbohydrates: 8 grams
Fat: less than 1 gram
Sodium: 21 milligrams

Spinach Soup

Makes 6 Cups

2 pounds fresh spinach
1/2 cup chopped onion
1/2 cup chopped cooked smoked turkey bacon
1 teaspoon crushed red pepper flakes

1 teaspoon ground celery powder
1 cup skim milk

1. Wash the spinach (make sure all the dirt and sand has been removed) and remove excess stems.
2. Place the spinach, onion, and turkey bacon in a food processor or blender and chop for 2 minutes.
3. In a large pot combine 4 cups of water, the red pepper, and ground celery. Bring to a boil and continue boiling for about 10 minutes. Add the spinach mixture and milk and cook another 15 minutes over medium heat.

Per Serving
Calories: 80
Protein: 8 grams
Carbohydrates: 11 grams
Fat: 2 grams
Sodium: 270 milligrams

Potato Carrot Soup
10 Servings

6 white potatoes, peeled and diced (about 7 cups)
2 cups carrots, peeled and diced
2 cups diced onions
1/2 teaspoon celery seeds
1/2 teaspoon dried marjoram
2-1/2 cups skim milk
1 teaspoon freshly ground black pepper
1/2 teaspoon crushed red pepper flakes

1. In a large pot, bring 6 cups of water to a boil. Add the potatoes, carrots, onions, celery seeds, and marjoram, and cook, covered, for about 20 minutes or until the vegetables are very soft. Drain the vegetables, careful to reserve about 4 cups of the liquid (this will be used as stock water later).
2. Put the vegetables in a food processor and mix until smooth.
3. Pour the milk and 3 cups of the reserved stock into a pot and bring to a boil. Add the vegetables along with the black pepper and crushed red pepper. Cook for about 5 minutes. Add more stock for a thinner soup.

Per Serving
Calories: 155
Protein: 6 grams
Carbohydrates: 33 grams
Fat: less than 1 gram
Sodium: 46 milligrams

Macaroni Salad

4 servings

3 cups cooked elbow macaroni
1/2 cup diced celery
1/2 cup diced dill pickle
3 tablespoons diced pimento
2 tablespoons diced onion
3 tablespoons nonfat plain yogurt
1 teaspoon chopped fresh dill
1/2 teaspoon ground red pepper

1. In a large bowl, mix the pasta, celery, pickle, pimento, and onion.
2. In a separate bowl, blend together the yogurt, dill, and pepper.
3. Add the dressing to the pasta and mix thoroughly. Chill in the refrigerator for about 3 hours, to allow flavors to develop before serving.

Per Serving
Calories: 150
Protein: 5 grams
Carbohydrates: 30 grams
Fat: 1 gram
Sodium: 77 milligrams

Classic Potato Salad

4 servings

3 cups of white potatoes, peeled, cooked, and cut into 1-inch cubes
1/2 cup chopped celery
1/2 cup sweet pickle relish
1/2 cup sliced scallions (green onions)
1 tablespoon balsamic vinegar
1 tablespoon finely chopped fresh dill
1-1/2 teaspoons Dijon mustard
1/2 teaspoon ground white pepper

1. In a large bowl, combine all the ingredients, mixing well. Chill in the refrigerator for at least 2 hours, to allow flavors to develop, before serving.

Per Serving
Calories: 180
Protein: 4 grams
Carbohydrates: 43 grams
Fat: less than 1 gram
Sodium: 199 milligrams

Cole Slaw

4 servings

2 cups shredded green cabbage
2 cups shredded red cabbage
1/2 cup shredded carrots
1/2 cup diced onion
1/2 cup diced sweet pickles
3 tablespoons nonfat plain yogurt
2 tablespoons sugar
2 tablespoons freshly squeezed lemon juice
1/2 teaspoon lemon zest (grated from the lemon peel)

1. Mix all the ingredients thoroughly in a large bowl.
2. Chill in the refrigerator for 2 to 3 hours before serving

Per Serving
Calories: 80
Protein: 2 grams
Carbohydrates: 20 grams
Fat: less than 1 gram
Sodium: 149 milligrams

String Bean Salad

6 servings

1 pound fresh string beans, steamed to desired tenderness
1/2 cup diced tomato
1/2 cup diced cucumber
1/2 cup diced green bell peppers
1/2 cup diced onion
3 tablespoons Dijon mustard
1 tablespoon balsamic vinegar

1. In a large bowl, combine the string beans, tomato, cucumber, bell pepper, and onion.
2. In a cup combine the mustard and vinegar. Pour the dressing over the vegetables and mix well.
3. Chill in the refrigerator for 1 to 2 hours to allow flavors to develop before serving.

Per Serving
Calories: 45
Protein: 2 grams
Carbohydrates: 9 grams
Fat: 1 gram
Sodium: 124 milligrams

Carrot Salad

6 servings

1 pound carrots, shredded
1/2 cup nonfat mayonnaise
1/2 cup dark raisins

1/2 cup golden raisins
1 tablespoon cider vinegar
1 tablespoon sugar

1. In a large bowl, combine all the ingredients and mix well. For a creamier texture, use more nonfat mayonnaise.
2. Chill in the refrigerator for 2 hours before serving

Per Serving
Calories: 130
Protein: 2 grams
Carbohydrates: 33 grams
Fat: less than 1 gram
Sodium: 196 milligrams

Cucumber Salad

4 servings

2-1/2 cups thinly sliced unpeeled cucumbers
1/2 cup cubed tomatoes
1 tablespoon chopped fresh Italian parsley
1 teaspoon chopped fresh tarragon
1/2 cup diced onion
2 tablespoons balsamic vinegar
1 teaspoon freshly ground black pepper

1. Combine the cucumbers, tomatoes, parsley, tarragon, and onion in a large bowl.
2. In a cup, combine the vinegar and pepper and pour over the salad.

3. Mix well and chill in the refrigerator for about 3 hours to allow flavors to develop before serving.

Per Serving
Calories: 25
Protein: 1 gram
Carbohydrates: 5 grams
Fat: less than 1 gram
Sodium: 5 milligrams

MAIN DISHES

Codfish Cakes

8 Servings

1 pound cod fillets, steamed
1 teaspoon lemon juice
1 cup mashed potatoes
2 cloves garlic, minced
1 tablespoon finely minced rosemary leaves
3 teaspoons olive oil
1 teaspoon salt
1 teaspoon Lemon Pepper
1/2 teaspoon dry mustard
2 tablespoons bread crumbs
2 tablespoons flour

1. Put steamed fish into a large mixing bowl, sprinkle on lemon juice and toss. Add potatoes and gently fold into the dish.
2. In a small saucepan, saute garlic and rosemary in 1 teaspoon oil over medium heat for 1 minute, until garlic is

lightly browned. Add garlic mixture, salt, lemon pepper, and mustard to the fish mixture and knead with your hands to mix thoroughly.

3. Shape into eight patties, and dredge in a combined mixture of bread crumbs and flour. Let chill in refrigerator for 1/2 hour.
4. In a large nonstick skillet, heat 1 teaspoon oil over medium-high heat. When hot, add four patties and cook for 3 minutes on each side, until well browned. Remove and drain on paper towels. Repeat with the remaining oil and patties.

Per Serving
Calories: 107
Carbohydrate: 8 grams
Fat: 3 grams
Sodium: 400 milligrams

Salmon Croquettes

8 servings

3 cloves garlic, minced
3 teaspoons olive oil
1 pound salmon fillet
1/2 cup dry vermouth
2 teaspoons butter
1 tablespoon flour
1/2 cup evaporated skim milk
1/2 cup mashed potatoes
1 teaspoon salt

2 teaspoons Lemon Pepper
2 tablespoons chopped parsley
2 tablespoons chopped chives
1 tablespoon chopped dill
1 egg, beaten
2 teaspoons lemon juice
1/2 cup flour
2 tablespoons bread crumbs

1. Saute garlic in 1 teaspoon oil and set aside.
2. Steam salmon in vermouth for 10 minutes, until firm, set aside to cool, and flake.
3. In a large saucepan, melt butter. When butter begins to bubble, stir in the flour. Slowly add the milk, stirring while pouring, until mixture is smooth and thickened. Add salmon, garlic, potatoes, salt, lemon pepper, parsley, chives, dill, egg, and lemon juice.
4. On a plate, combine flour and bread crumbs. Run hands under cold water and shape salmon into eight patties and dredge in flour mixture. Chill for at least 1/2 hour.
5. In a nonstick skillet or cast-iron skillet, heat 1 teaspoon oil. Place four patties in the pan and cook 3 minutes on each side, until well browned. Drain on paper towels. Add remaining oil to the pan and cook the remaining four patties.

Per Serving
Calories: 129
Carbohydrates: 11 grams
Fat: 4 grams
Sodium: 379 milligrams

Skinless Fried Chicken

6 servings

6 skinless, bone-in chicken breast halves
2 cups 1 percent fat buttermilk
1/2 teaspoon salt
1 teaspoon freshly ground pepper
1 tablespoon lemon juice
1 teaspoon Seasoned Salt
2 teaspoons ground sage
2 teaspoons paprika
1/2 cup finely ground cracker crumbs
1 teaspoon baking powder
1/2 cup olive oil
1 cup flour

1. Split each halved chicken breast in half again. Soak each chicken piece in the buttermilk for 1 hour. Remove chicken from buttermilk mixture and pat dry. Discard milk.
2. Place chicken on a plate and sprinkle with salt, pepper, and lemon juice. Toss to mix evenly. In a paper bag, combine the seasoned salt, sage, paprika, cracker crumbs, flour and baking powder; shake the bag to mix.
3. In a large cast-iron or nonstick skillet, heat the oil over medium-high heat. Dredge chicken in the flour mixture and shake off excess. When oil is very hot, lay the chicken pieces in the pan, fleshy side down, and immediately reduce heat to medium. Cook for 10-12 minutes and turn the chicken over to cook for another 8-10 minutes, until chicken is golden brown. Remove and drain on paper towels.

Per Serving
Calories: 308
Carbohydrates: 25 grams
Fat: 7 grams
Sodium: 487 milligrams

Grilled Barbecued Chicken

6 Servings

6 boneless, skinless chicken breast halves
1/2 teaspoon salt
1/2 teaspoon freshly ground pepper
1 cup Barbecue Sauce

1. Put chicken in a shallow dish and sprinkle with salt and pepper. Pour on barbecue sauce, toss well, and let sit in refrigerator for at least 2 hours. Discard sauce or use as a baste for immediate use only.
2. Preheat grill for 15 minutes. Put chicken pieces, fleshy side down, on the hot grill and cook for 10 minutes, until chicken is slightly charred. Turn over and cook for 10 minutes more, basting occasionally.

Per Serving
Calories: 204
Carbohydrates: 14 grams
Fat: 3 grams
Sodium: 421 milligrams

Barbecue Sauce
Makes 2 Cups

1 small onion, minced
3 cloves garlic, crushed
1 tablespoon butter
1 tablespoon finely minced gingerroot
1/2 cup dark brown sugar
1/2 cup tomato puree
2 tablespoons tomato paste
1/2 cup red wine
1/2 cup dark beer
1 tablespoon Worcestershire sauce
2 tablespoons balsamic vinegar
1 teaspoon Dijon mustard
1 teaspoon salt
1 teaspoon ground sage
1 teaspoon Lemon Pepper
3 sprigs of thyme
1 hot chili pepper, seeded and finely chopped
1/2 teaspoon ground cumin

In a 2-quart saucepan, saute onion and garlic in butter over medium heat. Add remaining ingredients, increase heat to high, and bring to a boil. Reduce heat to low and simmer for 25 minutes, until thickened.

Per Serving – 1 Tablespoon
Calories: 11
Fat: 1 gram

Carbohydrates: 1 gram
Sodium: 96 milligrams

Spinach, Chicken, and Rice

6 Servings

nonstick cooking spray
2 pounds boneless, skinless chicken breast, cut into 1-inch cubes
1 pound fresh spinach, rinsed and chopped
2 cups long-grain white rice
1 bay leaf
1 teaspoon fresh rosemary
2 teaspoons fresh dill
2 tablespoons fresh lemon juice
1 teaspoon freshly ground black pepper

1. In a nonstick skillet lightly coated with nonstick cooking spray, saute the chicken for about 10 minutes on medium heat or until lightly browned. Add the spinach and saute until it is completely wilted, stirring continuously.
2. Add the rice, the remaining ingredients, and 4 cups of water. Cover and cook over low heat for about 20 minutes.

Per Serving
Calories: 180
Protein: 21 grams
Carbohydrates: 19 grams
Fat: 2 grams
Sodium: 77 milligrams

Chicken with Cream Gravy

6 Servings

6 large, skinless, bone-in chicken breast halves
1 tablespoon lemon
1 teaspoon freshly ground white pepper
1/2 teaspoon paprika
2 teaspoons olive oil
1/2 cup flour
1 cup chicken stock
1 teaspoon arrowroot mixed with 1/2 cup hot water
2 cups evaporated skim milk, warmed
1/2 teaspoon mace
1/2 teaspoon ground sage
1 teaspoon salt
Pinch of cayenne

1. Split the halved chicken breasts in half again; place them in a shallow bowl and sprinkle with lemon juice, pepper, and paprika. Toss to mix.
2. In a large nonstick skillet, heat 1 teaspoon oil over medium-high heat. Dredge six chicken pieces in flour, shake off excess, and panfry for 3-5 minutes on each side, until well browned. Remove from pan and repeat with the remaining oil and chicken.
3. Add chicken stock to the pan and stir to loosen the browned bits from the pan. Pour in the arrowroot mixture and continue to stir for 2 minutes more, until mixture thickens. Add milk, mace, sage, salt, and cayenne and

reduce heat to low. Return chicken to pan and simmer for 30 minutes, covered, until chicken is tender.

Per Serving
Calories: 183
Carbohydrates: 10 grams
Fat: 3 grams
Sodium: 484 milligrams

Country Chicken with Cornmeal Waffles

6 servings

1 pound skinless, boneless chicken breasts
2 tablespoons dry sherry
1 tablespoon butter
1 tablespoon chopped shallots
1-1/2 tablespoons flour
2 cups evaporated skim milk
1/2 teaspoon salt
1 tablespoon chopped chives
1 teaspoon chopped dill
1 teaspoon grated lemon zest
1/2 teaspoon freshly ground white pepper
Cornmeal Waffles

1. Pound the chicken breasts flat with a heavy mallet. Heat a 13-inch nonstick saute pan over medium-high heat and sear the breasts for about 3 minutes on each side. Add the sherry, scraping up the browned bits with a wooden spoon. Remove the breasts from pan, let cool and mince.

2. In the same skillet, melt the butter and saute the shallots for about 1 minute. Add the flour and stir until the butter is absorbed into the flour. Add the milk slowly, stirring until the mixture thickens. (The mixture should be the consistency of a light soup.) Add more milk if a thinner sauce is desired.
3. Add the chicken cubes to the sauce, followed by the salt, chives, dill, and zest, and simmer for about 5 minutes. Remove from the heat and add the pepper. Serve over Cornmeal Waffles.

Cornmeal Waffles

6 waffles

1 cup all-purpose unbleached flour
1 cup cornmeal
2 teaspoons baking powder
1/2 teaspoon baking soda
2 tablespoons sugar
1/2 teaspoon salt
1 egg
2 cups evaporated skim milk
1 teaspoon olive oil
2 egg whites

1. Preheat the waffle iron. Sift together all the dry ingredients. Beat the egg and milk together and slowly pour the mixture into the dry ingredients. Stir in the oil.
2. Whip the egg whites until stiff and gently fold them into the batter. Lightly grease the waffle iron and drop the batter into the center of the iron. Cook according to manufacturer's instructions.

Per Serving
Calories: 327
Carbohydrates: 62 grams
Fat: 6 grams
Sodium: 546 milligrams

Stuffed Pork Tenderloin with Vegetables

4 to 6 Servings

1/2 cup diced broccoli stems
1/2 cup diced cauliflower florets
1/2 cup diced carrots
1 egg white, lightly beaten
1 tablespoon fresh lime juice, plus 1 teaspoon
1/2 teaspoon dried rubbed sage
2 lean pork tenderloins (about 2 pounds)
2 tablespoons minced fresh garlic
1 teaspoon freshly ground black pepper
nonstick cooking spray

1. Preheat oven to 400 F. In a bowl, mix the broccoli, cauliflower, carrots, egg white, lime juice, and sage. Set aside.
2. Along the length of each tenderloin, slice a pocket deep enough for half of the stuffing. Stuff each tenderloin with the stuffing, season them with garlic and pepper, and place them in a roasting pan lightly coated with cooking spray. Sprinkle some additional lime juice on top of the tenderloins and spray each with cooking spray.
3. Cover the pan tightly with foil and roast for about 1 hour turning the tenderloins halfway through cooking.

Per Serving
Calories: 215
Protein: 35 grams
Carbohydrates: 3 grams
Fat: 6 grams
Sodium: 121 milligrams

African-American Meatballs

Herbal Barbecue Sauce (recipe follows) is a tasty complement to these meatballs

Makes 12-15 1-1/2 inch meatballs

1 cup whole wheat bread crumbs (toast and crumble your own, store-bought are high in fat)
1 tablespoon minced onion
2 teaspoons freshly ground black pepper
1 pound ground turkey breast
3 egg whites, lightly beaten
3 tablespoons Louisiana Hot Sauce
2 tablespoons ketchup
1 teaspoon prepared horseradish
nonstick cooking spray

1. Mix the bread crumbs, onion, and black pepper together well in a large bowl. Add the ground turkey breast, egg whites, hot sauce, ketchup, and horseradish. Using your hands, mix thoroughly.

2. Cover the mixture with plastic wrap and refrigerate for 4 to 5 hours so that the flavors can blend. Shape the mixture into 12 to 15 1-1/2- inch balls.
3. Preheat oven to 375 F. Lightly coat a baking sheet with nonstick cooking spray. Place the meatballs on the baking sheet and bake for about 40 minutes or until the meatballs are firm and no longer pink on the inside.

Per Meatball
Calories: 50
Protein: 8 grams
Carbohydrates: 2 grams
Fat: 1 gram
Sodium: 63 milligrams

Herbal Barbecue Sauce

Makes about 2 cups

1 tablespoon finely chopped fresh marjoram
1 tablespoon finely chopped fresh rosemary
1 tablespoon finely chopped fresh sage
1/2 cup cider vinegar
1 teaspoon freshly ground black pepper
1/2 cup ketchup
1/2 cup water
1/3 cup honey
1 teaspoon mustard powder

Combine all the ingredients in a small saucepan and bring to a boil, stirring constantly. Reduce heat and simmer for about 5 minutes.

Per 2 Tablespoons
Calories: 31
Protein: 0 grams
Carbohydrates: 8 grams
Fat: less than 1 gram
Sodium: 102 milligrams

Smothered Cabbage with Smoked Turkey

6 Servings

5 cups chopped cabbage
1 cup smoked skinless turkey breast, chopped
1/2 cup sliced carrot
1 tablespoon balsamic vinegar
1 tablespoon sugar
1 teaspoon ground white pepper

1. Pour 2 cups of water in a large skillet and bring to a boil. Add the cabbage, turkey, carrots, vinegar, sugar, and pepper. Cover the pan and cook for about 1 hour over a low-medium heat, stirring occasionally.
2. Do not let all of the water evaporate from the pan; add more if needed so that the cabbage does not burn.

Per Serving
Calories: 75
Protein: 12 grams
Carbohydrates: 6 grams
Fat: less than 1 gram
Sodium: 34 milligrams

SIDE DISHES

Red Beans and Rice

8 Servings

2 cups dried kidney beans
1 pound skinless smoked turkey breast, cut up in cubes
1 cup chopped onion
1 tablespoon minced fresh garlic
1 tablespoon Soul Food Seasoning (under section entitled "Extras")
1 teaspoon celery seeds
1 bay leaf
2 cups long-grain white rice

1. Sort and rinse the beans. Place the beans in a pot with the turkey breast, and add enough water to cover completely. Bring to a boil, then reduce the heat to low; cover and simmer for about 2 hours.
2. Add the onion, garlic, Soul Food Seasoning, celery seeds, and bay leaf and cook for an additional 45 minutes.
3. In a separate pot, bring 5 cups of water to a boil. Add the rice, cover, reduce heat, and simmer for about 20 minutes. Serve the beans over the rice or combine rice and beans together in a large serving bowl.

Per Serving
Calories: 260
Protein: 26 milligrams
Carbohydrates: 35 grams
Fat: 1 gram
Sodium: 38 milligrams

Mississippi Dirty Rice

4 Servings

1 cup brown rice
1/2 cup ground all-white turkey
1/2 cup diced onion
2 tablespoons diced green bell pepper
1 tablespoon Soul Food Seasoning (under section entitled, "Extras")
1 teaspoon chopped fresh garlic
1 teaspoon freshly ground black pepper
nonstick cooking spray

1. Bring 3 cups of water to a boil in a medium saucepan and add the rice. Cover and cook for about 50 minutes over a low-medium heat; set aside.
2. Saute the ground turkey, onion, green pepper, Soul Food Seasoning, garlic, and black pepper in a nonstick skillet lightly coated with nonstick cooking spray for about 15 minutes over a low heat.
3. In a large bowl, stir together the rice and turkey mixture.

Per Serving
Calories: 160
Protein: 9 grams
Carbohydrates: 26 grams
Fat: 2 grams
Sodium: 26 milligrams

Macaroni and Cheese

6 Servings

2 cups elbow macaroni

1/2 cup grated reduced-fat cheddar cheese

1/3 cup skim milk

2 tablespoons sliced scallions

1 egg white, lightly beaten

1 tablespoons nonfat Parmesan cheese topping

1. Cook the macaroni according to package instructions, and drain.
2. Place the macaroni in a large bowl and add the cheddar cheese, milk, scallions, and egg white. Stir well.
3. Preheat oven to 375 F. Place the macaroni in a nonstick casserole pan and sprinkle the Parmesan cheese on top. Bake about 25 minutes or until the top is browned and firm.

Per Serving

Calories: 155

Protein: 9 grams

Carbohydrates: 27 grams

Fat: less than 1 gram

Sodium: 115 milligrams

Cream-Like Potatoes

4 servings

2 pounds white potatoes

1/2 cup plain nonfat yogurt

1/2 cup skim milk

2 tablespoons Dijon mustard
1 teaspoon ground white pepper
1 teaspoon fresh lemon juice
1 tablespoon nonfat Parmesan cheese topping

1. Peel the potatoes and cut them into quarters. Rinse well. Cook them in boiling water for about 20 minutes or until fork-tender. Drain the potatoes and place in a large bowl.
2. Add the yogurt, milk, Dijon, pepper, and lemon juice. Mash well with a potato masher, leaving no lumps. For a drier or creamier texture, adjust the amount of milk.
3. Sprinkle the Parmesan cheese on top of the potatoes and serve.

Per Serving
Calories: 245
Protein: 8 grams
Carbohydrates: 52 grams
Fat: 1 gram
Sodium: 250 milligrams

Scalloped Potatoes

6 servings

1 cup skim milk
3 cups peeled white potatoes, thinly sliced
1/2 cup sliced white button mushrooms
2 tablespoons finely chopped fresh parsley
2 tablespoons finely chopped onion
2 tablespoons finely chopped scallions

1 tablespoon fresh lemon juice
1 teaspoon ground white pepper

1. Heat the skim milk in a large skillet for about 3 minutes. Add the potatoes and mushrooms, and cook on a low heat for 20 minutes or until the texture becomes soft. Stir constantly to avoid sticking or burning, but be careful not to break potato slices.
2. Add the parsley, onions, scallions, lemon juice, and white pepper. Cook another 5 minutes, stirring frequently.

Per Serving
Calories: 70
Protein: 3 grams
Carbohydrates: 15 grams
Fat: less than 1 gram
Sodium: 25 milligrams

Homemade Fries

4 servings

nonstick cooking spray
2 pounds Idaho potatoes
3 egg whites, slightly beaten
1/2 cup all-purpose flour
2 tablespoons Soul Food Seasoning (under section entitled, "Extras")
1/2 teaspoon crushed celery seeds

1. Preheat oven to 400 F. Lightly coat a baking sheet with cooking spray. Peel the potatoes, cut them lengthwise into

about 1/2-inch-thick sticks, and place them in a large bowl. Pour the egg whites over them and toss to coat all the potato slices.

2. Combine the flour, Soul Food Seasoning, and celery seeds in a plastic bag. Remove about one handful of potatoes from the bowl and drain off any excess egg white. Put the potatoes in the bag and shake well to coat the potatoes. Remove the potatoes from the bag and spread them on the baking sheet. Repeat until all the potatoes are coated.
3. Spray the potatoes with cooking spray. Bake for 40 minutes or until the fries are crispy, turning them every 10 minutes with a spatula, so that they are brown and crispy all over.

Per Serving
Calories: 145
Protein: 6 grams
Carbohydrates: 29 grams
Fat: less than 1 gram
Sodium: 55 milligrams

Mushroom Rice

4 servings

1 cup long-grain rice
nonstick cooking spray
1-1/2 cups chopped Portabello mushrooms
1/2 cup chopped scallions
2 tablespoons fresh lemon juice
1 tablespoon finely chopped fresh marjoram
1 tablespoon finely chopped fresh parsley

1 teaspoon ground white pepper
1 teaspoon Soul Food Seasoning (under section entitled, "Extras")

1. Pour the rice in a saucepan sprayed with nonstick cooking spray and cook stirring frequently on a low heat for about 3 minutes. Add 3 cups of water and the mushrooms. Cover and cook for about 20 minutes on a low heat or until all the liquid has been absorbed and the rice is tender.
2. Stir in the scallions, lemon juice, marjoram, parsley, white pepper, and Soul Food Seasoning. Let stand, covered, for 3 to 5 minutes before serving.

Per Serving
Calories: 70
Protein: 2 grams
Carbohydrates: 15 grams
Fat: 1 gram
Sodium: 8 milligrams

Green Onion and Cheese Grits

8 servings

1 tablespoon butter
4 cups water
1/2 teaspoon salt
1 cup grits
1/2 cup chopped scallions, green and white parts
1/2 cup freshly grated Parmesan cheese

1. In a 2-quart saucepan, bring water to a boil over high heat. Sprinkle grits in by the tablespoon, stirring vigorously to avoid clotting. Reduce heat to low and simmer 15 minutes, continuing to stir until grits become creamy and thick.
2. Remove from heat and immediately pour into a lightly buttered serving dish. Sprinkle scallions and cheese on top and serve.

Per Serving
Calories: 98
Carbohydrates: 16 grams
Fat: 2 grams
Sodium: 195 milligrams

Baked Cheese Grits

4 Servings

1 cup uncooked grits
1/2 teaspoon reduced-fat margarine
3 egg whites, lightly beaten
1/2 cup grated reduced-fat cheddar cheese
1 teaspoon finely minced garlic

1. Preheat oven to 350 F. Bring 4 cups of water to a boil in a medium saucepan over high heat. Stir in the grits and reduce heat, cooking until they become thick, about 10 minutes.
2. Stir in the margarine, egg whites, cheese, and garlic, mixing thoroughly. Pour the mixture into a 9-inch nonstick pie pan and bake 40 to 50 minutes, or until lightly browned on

the top. Remove from oven and cool in pan on wire rack. When grits cool, cut into small squares.

Per Serving
Calories: 75
Protein: 6 grams
Carbohydrates: 9 grams
Fat: 2 grams
Sodium: 234 milligrams

Unfried Hush Puppies

Makes 18 Hush Puppies

Nonstick cooking spray
1-1/2 cups yellow cornmeal
1/2 cup self-rising flour
2-1/2 teaspoons baking powder
1 tablespoon sugar
1/2 teaspoon salt
1/2 cup chopped onion
2 tablespoons chopped fresh parsley
2 cups skim milk
1 egg white, lightly beaten
1/2 cup water

1. Preheat oven to 400 F. Lightly coat an 18-cup muffin pan with nonstick cooking spray. Mix the cornmeal, flour, baking powder, sugar, and salt together. Fold in the onion, parsley, milk, egg white, and water. Pour the batter into the prepared muffin pan filling each 1/2 full. Bake 20-25 minutes or until golden brown.

Per Serving
Calories: 60
Protein: 2 grams
Carbohydrates: 12 grams
Fat: less than 1 gram
Sodium: 272 milligrams

Jalapeno Corn Bread

6 Servings

nonstick cooking spray
2 cups yellow cornmeal
1 cup all-purpose flour
2-1/2 teaspoons baking powder
1 tablespoon sugar
2 diced fresh jalapeno peppers, seeded and chopped
1 cup skim milk
6 egg whites
1/2 cup cider vinegar

1. Preheat oven to 375 F. Lightly coat a 9-1/2 x 9-1/2-inch baking pan or 12-cup muffin pan with nonstick cooking spray. Mix the cornmeal, flour, baking powder, and sugar together in a large bowl. Add the peppers, milk, egg whites, and vinegar. Stir with a spoon until thoroughly mixed.
2. Spoon the batter into the prepared pan. Bake 45 to 50 minutes or until the top of the corn bread is firm and light brown on the top. Cool in pan on wire rack.

Per Serving
Calories: 200
Protein: 8 grams
Carbohydrates: 39 grams
Fat: 1 gram
Sodium: 130 milligrams

Sweet Potato Biscuits

Makes about 14

Nonstick cooking spray
2 cups all-purpose flour
2 teaspoons baking powder
1 tablespoon granulated sugar
1/2 teaspoon salt
1 tablespoon reduced-fat margarine
1 cup mashed sweet potato
1/2 teaspoon ground cinnamon
1/2 teaspoon grated nutmeg
1 cup skim milk
1 egg white

1. Preheat oven to 400 F. Lightly coat a baking sheet with nonstick cooking spray. Using an electric mixer, combine the flour, baking powder, sugar, salt, and margarine. Then slowly mix in the sweet potatoes, cinnamon, nutmeg, and milk. Stir in the egg white.
2. On a lightly floured board, roll the dough out to 1/2-inch thickness. Using a biscuit cutter, cut the dough into 2-inch circles and place them on the baking sheet. Bake about 25 minutes or until they are firm in the center.

Per Serving
Calories: 100
Protein: 3 grams
Carbohydrates: 20 grams
Fat: less than 1 gram
Sodium: 290 milligrams

Mashed Potatoes

8 servings

8 large potatoes, scrubbed
1 tablespoon butter
2 tablespoons minced chives
1/2 cup 1 percent fat buttermilk, warmed
2 tablespoons reduced-fat mayonnaise
1 teaspoon salt
Freshly ground white pepper

1. Boil potatoes in water to cover for 20 to 25 minutes, or until tender when a fork is inserted. When fairly cool, drain and grate, or put through a potato ricer, including the skins, into a large bowl.
2. Add butter and chives, and mash. With a large fork, whip the potatoes while adding buttermilk. Add mayonnaise, salt, and pepper, and whip again.

Per Serving
Calories: 119
Carbohydrates: 21 grams
Fat: 2 grams
Sodium: 306 milligrams

VEGETABLES

String Beans with Potatoes

8 servings

1 tablespoon olive oil
1 whole onion
1 pound green beans, trimmed
1 pound red new potatoes, quartered
1 teaspoon salt
1/2 teaspoon grated lemon zest
1 tablespoon lemon juice
1/2 teaspoon freshly ground white pepper

1. Heat olive oil in large heavy skillet. Saute onion in oil for 15 minutes, until golden.
2. Blanch beans for 5 minutes in boiling water, then plunge into a bowl of ice water. Drain.
3. Add beans to the onion mixture in the skillet, and add potatoes, salt, and lemon zest. Cook over medium heat for 30 minutes, or until potatoes are soft. Add lemon juice and pepper.

Per Serving
Calories: 81
Carbohydrates: 15 grams
Fat: 1 gram
Sodium: 342 milligrams

Mashed Yams

6 servings

6 large yams
1 tablespoon butter
1/2 cup evaporated skim milk
1/8 cup lime juice
1 tablespoon dark rum
1 teaspoon coconut milk
1 tablespoon maple syrup
1/2 teaspoon cinnamon
1/2 teaspoon allspice
1/2 teaspoon nutmeg
1/2 teaspoon ground cloves
1/2 teaspoon salt
1 tablespoon freshly ground white pepper
1/4 teaspoon cayenne

1. In water to cover, boil the yams in their skins for 45 minutes, or until soft when a fork is inserted.
2. Cool, peel, and cube yams. Add butter, milk, lime juice, rum, coconut milk, and syrup and mash. Add cinnamon, allspice, nutmeg, cloves, salt, pepper, and cayenne and whip until smooth.

Per Serving
Calories: 222
Carbohydrates: 46 grams
Fat: 2 grams
Sodium: 217 milligrams

Fried Green Tomatoes

4 servings

6 large green tomatoes (about 3 pounds)
2 tablespoons lemon juice
1/2 cup cornmeal
2 teaspoons freshly ground black pepper
nonstick cooking spray

1. Slice each tomato into 1/2-inch-thick slices. Sprinkle the lemon juice on the tomatoes.
2. Mix the cornmeal and black pepper in a plastic bag. Put the tomato slices into the bag and shake well.
3. Coat a cast-iron skillet or nonstick saute pan with nonstick cooking spray. Fry the tomatoes, over medium-high heat, until they are light brown on each side.

Per Serving
Calories: 105
Protein: 3 grams
Carbohydrates: 22 grams
Fat: 2 grams
Sodium: 22 milligrams

Black-Eyed Peas

8–10 Servings

3 cups dried black-eyed peas
1 cup chopped skinless smoked turkey breast
1 cup chopped onion
1/2 cup chopped carrot

1/2 cup chopped celery
2 tablespoons cider vinegar
2 tablespoons Soul Food Seasoning (under section entitled, "Extras")
1 teaspoon fresh ground black pepper

1. Rinse and sort the peas. Place them in a large pot with enough water to cover and bring to boil. Once boiling, remove the pot from the heat, cover, and let stand for 1-1/2 hours.
2. Add the remaining ingredients and additional water if necessary to cover the peas. Place a lid on the pot, and cook on a low-medium heat for 1 hour, or until the peas are tender. Make sure there is enough water added in the pot to cover the peas throughout the cooking time.

Per Serving
Calories: 95
Protein: 9 grams
Carbohydrates: 14 grams
Fat: less than 1 gram
Sodium: 28 milligrams

Collard Greens

8 Servings

3 pounds collard greens, rinsed and chopped
1/2 pound smoked turkey breast, cubed
1 cup nonfat chicken broth
1/2 cup minced onion
1 teaspoon crushed red pepper flakes

1 teaspoon minced celery
1 teaspoon freshly ground black pepper

1. Place the collard greens and turkey in a large pot. Cover them with water, and cook on a medium heat, covered, for 20 minutes.
2. Add the chicken broth, onion, red pepper flakes, celery, and black pepper, and cook on a low-medium heat, covered, for about 45 minutes.

Per Serving
Calories: 95
Protein: 11 grams
Carbohydrates: 13 grams
Fat: 1 gram
Sodium: 78 milligrams

Honey Glazed Carrots

6 servings

1-1/2 pounds baby carrots
1 teaspoon ground coriander
1 tablespoon chopped fresh cilantro
1/2 cup honey

1. Wash and scrub the carrots. Place them in a saucepan with about 5 cups of water and heat to a boil. Cook the carrots for about 20 minutes over medium heat (do not overcook; the texture of the carrots should be slightly firm).

2. Preheat oven to 375F. Drain and place carrots in a casserole dish. Sprinkle the coriander and cilantro and pour the honey over the carrots.
3. Bake about 15 minutes or until the carrots are soft and slightly brown in color.

Per Serving
Calories: 100
Protein: 1 gram
Carbohydrates: 24 grams
Fat: less than 1 gram
Sodium: 27 milligrams

Fresh Fried Corn

4 servings

3 cups fresh corn cut from the cob
1/2 cup diced green bell pepper
2 tablespoons skim milk
1 tablespoon all-purpose flour
1 teaspoon minced fresh garlic
1 teaspoon ground white pepper
1/2 teaspoon paprika
nonstick cooking spray

1. Combine the corn, green pepper, milk, flour, garlic, white pepper, and paprika in a large skillet lightly coated with cooking spray.
2. Cook for about 15 minutes over low-medium heat, stirring constantly, to avoid sticking.

Per Serving
Calories: 120
Protein: 4 grams
Carbohydrates: 29 grams
Fat: less than 1 gram
Sodium: 11 milligrams

Fried Yellow Squash with Zucchini

6 servings

nonstick cooking spray
1 pound yellow squash, sliced 1/2-inch thick
1 pound zucchini, sliced 1/2-inch thick
1 cup chopped onion
1 cup chopped white mushrooms
1/2 pound smoked skinless turkey breast, chopped
1 teaspoon chopped fresh parsley
1 teaspoon Soul Food Seasoning (under section entitled, "Extras")
1 teaspoon freshly ground black pepper

1. Heat a large nonstick frying pan sprayed with cooking spray and cook the yellow squash, zucchini, onion, and mushrooms over low heat, covered, for about 15 minutes.
2. Add the turkey, parsley, Soul Food Seasoning, and black pepper, and continue to cook for about 30 minutes or until the vegetables are tender. Keep covered so that the juices from the vegetables do not evaporate.

Per Serving
Calories: 110
Protein: 18 grams
Carbohydrates: 9 grams
Fat: 1 gram
Sodium: 35 milligrams

Baked Lima Beans

10 servings

3 cups dried lima beans
1/3 pound skinless smoked turkey breast
1 cup nonfat canned chicken broth
1/2 cup diced onions
1/3 cup diced carrots
1 tablespoon minced fresh garlic
1 tablespoon Soul Food Seasoning (under section entitled, "Extras")
1 teaspoon freshly ground black pepper
1 bay leaf

1. Place the lima beans in a Dutch oven or large pot, and cover them with water. Let them soak for 3 hours at room temperature. Drain the water, sort the beans, rinse them thoroughly, and place them back in the Dutch oven.
2. Preheat oven to 350F. Add the turkey, chicken stock, onion, carrots, garlic, Soul Food Seasoning, pepper, and bay leaf to the beans. Add enough water to cover the beans by about 2 inches.
3. Cover and bake for about 4 hours. Make sure water is on top of the beans throughout the cooking time; if not, add

more water. When done, the beans should be tender – do not overcook.

Per Serving
Calories: 90
Protein: 8 grams
Carbohydrates: 15 grams
Fat: less than 1 gram
Sodium: 47 milligrams

Pickled Okra

1 quart
1 pound fresh okra (about 8 to 10 pieces)
2 cloves garlic, peeled
2 cups distilled white vinegar
1 sprig fresh dill
2 jalapeno peppers

1. Wash and dry the okra. Place the garlic in a sterilized one-quart canning jar.
2. In a saucepan over high heat, bring the vinegar to boiling. Pour the hot vinegar over the okra in the jar. Put the dill and jalapeno peppers in the jar and let cool until it reaches room temperature.
3. Seal the jar with a clean sterilized lid. Let the jar set for 4 to 5 weeks in the refrigerator before opening and eating.

Per Serving
Calories: 25
Protein: 1 gram
Carbohydrates: 6 grams
Fat: less than 1 gram
Sodium: 18 milligrams

DESSERTS

Deep-Dish Apple Pie

8 servings

10 large tart apples
Juice of 1 lemon
1/2 cup sugar
2 tablespoons Pie Spice (see recipe in this section)
1/2 teaspoon grated lemon zest
1 teaspoon finely chopped crystallized ginger
2 tablespoons ground tapioca
3 teaspoons butter
1 9-inch piecrust
Milk

1. Preheat the oven to 325 F. Butter a 9-inch deep-dish pie plate and set aside. Peel, core, and quarter the apples. Slice the apples 1/8 inch thick and place them in a large bowl of water mixed with the lemon juice.
2. In a small bowl, combine the sugar, pie spice, zest, ginger, and tapioca. Divide into three parts. Drain the apples and divide into thirds.

3. Place the first layer of apples in the baking dish, overlapping the apples if necessary. Sprinkle one third of the spice mixture evenly over the apples and top with 1 teaspoon butter. Repeat with a second and third layer.
4. Cover with the piecrust dough. Crimp the edges with a fork dipped in milk, and cut three slits in the top. Bake for 40 minutes, until golden brown on top. Let come to room temperature before slicing.

Per Serving
Calories: 289
Carbohydrates: 55 grams
Fat: 8 grams
Sodium: 159 milligrams

9-Inch Piecrust

1 cup all-purpose unbleached flour
1/2 teaspoon salt
1 teaspoon sugar
1/2 cup sweet butter, chilled
3 tablespoons nonfat sour cream, or 1 percent fat buttermilk, chilled
1 teaspoon ice water

1. Sift the flour, salt, and sugar into a large mixing bowl. Cut the butter into small chunks and, using your fingers, briskly rub the butter into the flour. (This step requires a bit of speed; otherwise, you'll end up with an oily crust.)
2. When the mixture resembles coarse meal, add the sour cream. Using a fork, work the sour cream into the meal.

Add ice water and pull the mixture together to form a ball. Knead the dough lightly two to three times. Reshape the dough into a ball again, wrap in plastic, and refrigerate for at least 1 hour.

3. Turn the ball out onto a lightly floured surface and roll out to the desired diameter (9 inches).

Note: For a prebaked pie shall, preheat the oven to 375 degrees F. Prick the crust with a fork and bake for 10 to 12 minutes, until golden. Cool.

Per Serving
Calories: 105
Carbohydrates: 12 grams
Fat: 5 grams
Sodium: 139 milligrams

Deep Dish Cherry Pie

8 servings

1 teaspoon butter
6 cups tart cherries, pitted and halved
1 cup sugar
2 teaspoons Pie Spice (see following recipe)
1/2 cup ground tapioca
1/2 teaspoon almond extract
1-9 inch piecrust
milk

1. Preheat the oven to 325 F. Butter a 9-inch deep-dish pie plate and set aside. Melt butter in a 3-quart saucepan over medium heat. Add cherries, sugar, pie spice, and tapioca,

and bring to a boil, stirring as it thickens, about 5 minutes. Remove from heat and stir in the almond extract. Pour cherry mixture into the baking dish. Place piecrust over cherries and crimp edges with a fork dipped in milk. Make three slits in the crust and bake for 30 minutes, until browned evenly on top. Serve at room temperature.

Per Serving
Calories: 272
Carbohydrates: 54 grams
Fat: 7 grams
Sodium: 146 milligrams

Pie Spice

Makes 2 teaspoons

1/2 teaspoon cinnamon
1/2 teaspoon nutmeg
1/2 teaspoon allspice
1/2 teaspoon ground cloves
1/2 teaspoon ground ginger
1/8 teaspoon ground cardamom
1/8 teaspoon freshly ground white pepper

Mix all ingredients together in a jar with a tight-fitting lid and store in a cool dry place. Shake before using.

Ambrosia

6 servings

4 oranges
2 bananas
1 small pineapple
1/2 cup freshly grated coconut meat
1/2 cup confectioners' sugar
2 tablespoons sweet sherry or kirsch

1. Peel and segment oranges. Slice the bananas crosswise 1/2 inch thick. Peel and core pineapple and cut into 1/2-inch cubes.
2. Place the oranges, bananas, and pineapple in a large bowl; add coconut, sugar, and sherry, and toss.

Per Serving
Calories: 255
Carbohydrates: 63 grams
Fat: 3 grams
Sodium: 9 milligrams

Lemon Pound Cake

12 servings

1 cup sugar
1 cup unsweetened applesauce
4 egg whites, at room temperature
2 tablespoons lemon extract
3 cups all-purpose flour
1/2 cup skim milk

1-1/2 teaspoons baking powder
2 teaspoons lemon zest
1/2 cup all-natural lemon preserves (no sugar added)
nonstick cooking spray

1. Preheat oven to 350F. With an electric mixer, beat the sugar and applesauce. Mix in the egg whites and lemon extract. Add the flour and milk alternately, using the flour first and last. Mix in the baking powder.
2. Pour the cake batter into a 10-inch tube pan (or one sprayed with cooking spray) and bake about 1-1/2 hours. Remove the cake from the pan and let it cool for about 20 minutes. Heat the 1/2 cup of lemon preserves in a saucepan for about 1 minute (until melted enough to pour) and drizzle over the cake.

Per Serving
Calories: 215
Protein: 4 grams
Carbohydrates: 29 grams
Fat: less than 1 gram
Sodium: 56 milligrams

Jelly Cake
12 servings

1 cup sugar
1/2 cup mashed banana
2-1/2 cups all-purpose flour
1 teaspoon baking powder
2 teaspoons vanilla extract

6 egg whites
nonstick cooking spray
1/2 cup all-natural raspberry preserves (no sugar added)

1. Preheat oven to 350F. In a large bowl, cream the sugar and banana with an electric mixer. Then slowly mix in the flour, baking powder, and vanilla extract. Mix in the egg whites one at a time.
2. Pour the cake batter into a nonstick 10-inch tube pan (or one sprayed with cooking spray) and bake about 1 hour or until an inserted toothpick comes out clean.
3. Let cool for 20 minutes, then remove the cake from the pan. In a saucepan, over low heat, heat the preserves until melted enough to pour, stirring constantly about one minute. Drizzle the preserves over the cake and serve.

Per Serving
Calories: 210
Protein: 4 grams
Carbohydrates: 47 grams
Fat: less than 1 gram
Sodium: 57 milligrams

Banana Pudding

8 servings

1/2 cup sugar
2 tablespoons cornstarch
2 cups evaporated skim milk
2 teaspoons vanilla extract

2-1/2 cups vanilla wafer crumbs
3 cups bananas, sliced
3 large egg whites, at room temperature
ground cinnamon

1. Preheat oven to 400F. Combine the sugar, cornstarch, and milk in a medium saucepan. Cook over a low heat, stirring constantly until the mixture thickens like pudding. Add the vanilla extract.
2. In a 9-inch or 10-inch casserole dish, arrange a layer of vanilla wafers (touching each other). Arrange a layer of banana slices on top of the wafers. Repeat with wafers and bananas.
3. Pour the thickened pudding mixture over the bananas. Using an electric mixer, beat the egg whites until stiff, then spread on top of the pudding. Sprinkle cinnamon on top.
4. Bake the pudding until the surface of the egg whites begins to brown. Let the custard cool for about 2 hours before serving.

Per Serving
Calories: 200
Protein: 7 Grams
Carbohydrates: 35 grams
Fat: 4 grams
Sodium: 129 milligrams

EXTRAS

Soul Food Seasoning

2 tablespoons ground red pepper flakes
2 tablespoons garlic powder
2 tablespoons onion powder
2 tablespoons dark chili powder
1 tablespoon paprika
1 teaspoon thyme powder
1 teaspoon freshly ground black pepper

Mix all the ingredients together. Store in a sealed container.

Index

Note: page numbers in **bold** refer to a diagram or table

About the Authors

Hilton M. Hudson II, M.D., F.A.C.S. is a practicing cardiac surgeon and the Clinical Director of Cardiothoracic Surgery at Rockford Health Systems, Rockford, IL. He graduated cum laude from Wabash College, and received his medical training at Indiana University Medical School. He trained in general surgery at Boston City Hospital and Boston University Hospital, Boston, MA. He did his cardiothoracic training at Ohio State University. Dr. Hudson is certified in both thoracic-cardiac surgery and general surgery. He is a diplomate of the American Board of Thoracic Surgery, a Fellow of the American College of Surgeons, and a Fellow of the College of Chest Physicians. He belongs to the American Medical Association, the National Medical Association, Boston Surgical Society, Hinton-Wright Society at Harvard Medical School, and the Zollinger Surgical Society.

Herbert Stern, Ph.D. is the retired Milligan Professor of English at Wabash College He has published widely on social and literary topics. He lives in Somerville, MA.